My Father's Legacy

The Story of

Doctor Nils August Johanson

Founder of Swedish Medical Center

Katharine Johanson Nordstrom

with Margaret Marshall

Library of Congress Control Number: 2002103206

ISBN 0-295-98265-9

Distributed by University of Washington Press,
P.O. Box 50096, Seattle, WA 98145-5096
www.washington.edu/uwpress

DEDICATION

I dedicate this book to my sons, John Nils and James Frederick Nordstrom, who through their leadership of the Nordstrom enterprises are continuing in the example of excellence set for them by their father and their two grandfathers.

My sons are fortunate to own an autobiography written many years ago by their paternal grandfather, John W. Nordstrom, who came to this country from Sweden at the age of 15. Through his diligence and industry he founded the store which was the forerunner of the national Nordstrom enterprises.

I have written this book so that my sons and their families would have a record of their maternal grandfather, also a Swedish immigrant, who made an invaluable contribution to the community. He was my father, Doctor Nils August Johanson. After arriving from Sweden as a young man, through hard work and sacrifice he obtained a medical education and came to Seattle as a surgeon. In 1910 he founded The Swedish Hospital, which has become a major medical center with an international reputation for the quality of its care and its leadership in the fight against cancer.

FOREWORD

Our family feels very fortunate that my mother was able to complete this memoir of her father before she passed away in June of 1999. We have elected to publish it just as she wrote it in 1995, rather than update it to show changes which have taken place with regard to our family members and the continuing progress of both the Swedish Medical Center and Nordstrom. While my father and my brother Jim did not live to see this book in published form, I'm glad they both had the opportunity to read the manuscript at the time it was completed.

John Nils Nordstrom
August 2001

ACKNOWLEDGMENTS

I would like to express my thanks to the following persons:

...To my beloved husband, Elmer Nordstrom, for the loving support he gave me, and for the important role he played in the development of the Swedish Medical Center.

...To all of those quoted in the book, for sharing their memories of my father.

...To staff members of the Swedish Medical Center, for their cooperation in locating archival material.

...To Margaret Marshall, for her valued assistance in the writing of this book.

CONTENTS

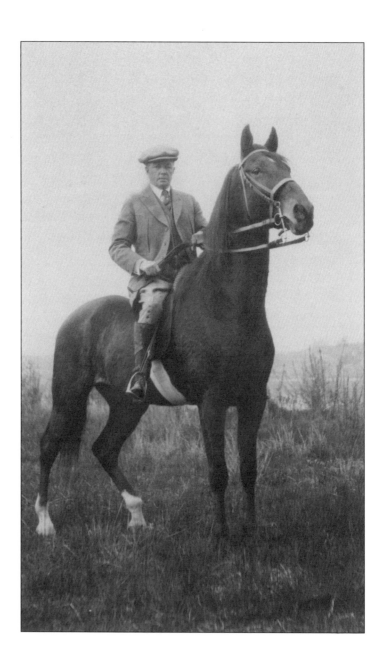

Chapter One

Voyage to a New Land

I have a favorite memory picture of my father as he was when I was about nine years old. It's a lovely fall day and he and I are astride our favorite horses, cantering briskly along a wooded path of the Olympic Riding Academy in Seattle. We both loved riding, and we thoroughly enjoyed one another's company. To everyone else he was Doctor Nils August Johanson, skilled surgeon and busy administrator of Swedish Hospital, but to me he was a loving father who found time in his crowded schedule to share a favorite pastime with his only child.

My father's childhood was not as privileged as mine. He was born in Lund, Sweden, on July 21, 1872, to Johan and Anna Johanson and was one of seven children. His brothers were Johan and Erik, and his four sisters were Beata (Ata), Anna, Henrika (Rika) and Eva. On the income his father earned as a tailor there probably were few luxuries.

Lund was a college town, at the southernmost tip of

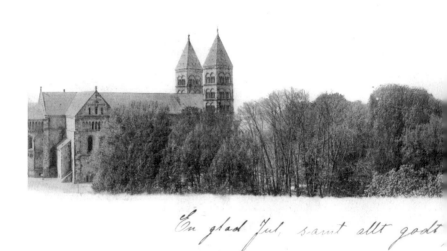

En glad Jul, samt allt godt

Above: Lund Sweden, the college town where my father was born.
Left to right; My father's parents: Johan and Anna Johanson. His sisters; Beata (Ata), Anna, Henrika (Rika), and Eva. My father, after he arrived in the United States. Wasn't he a handsome young fellow?

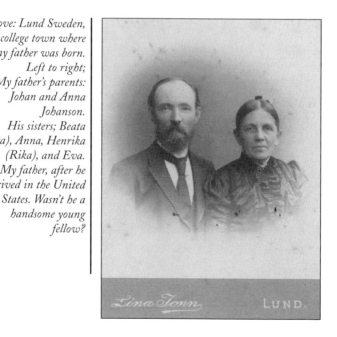

Lina Tonn   LUND.

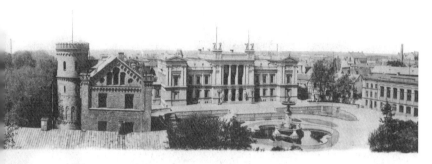

på det nya året önskas eder från hemm

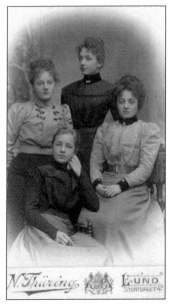

N. Thüring LUND STORTORGET 4

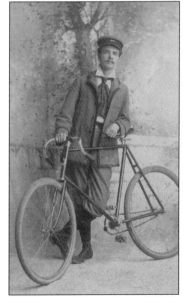

Sweden, and there was a medical school at the University. As Nils reached the teen years and began to think of what his future livelihood might be, he pictured himself not as a tailor like his father, but instead as a medical student at the University of Lund, preparing to be a doctor. It could only be a dream for him, however. The economy of Sweden had been at low ebb for a very long time. During the years my father was growing up, the only hope a young man had of bettering himself was to leave Sweden and journey to America. That was a step which took not only a great deal of courage, but also an outlay of hard cash to obtain even the steerage passage by which most emigrants left Sweden.

A younger brother, Erik, had somehow managed to scrape together enough money to get to the United States, and was working in Denver, Colorado. Many of those who emigrated wrote letters home painting a picture of comparative affluence. Encouraging reports received from Erik may have inspired in his brother a great desire to go to America himself. Young Nils perhaps reasoned that in such a wealthy country it might even be possible for someone like himself to fulfill his dream of becoming a doctor. If he remained in Sweden, there certainly was no chance at all of achieving that goal.

I don't know how my father managed to raise the money for his journey to the new world. Perhaps his parents scrimped and saved. His brother may have sent money from America. Nils probably worked very hard at some menial task until the magic day came when he had enough money to pay for the ocean voyage. A friend, a young man named J. Wiemer, had agreed to accompany him. One can imagine the excitement of the two young men when the time came to say farewell to family and friends and embark on a daring adventure. The year was 1893.

The United States experienced boom years during the early 1880's, making the promise of a new life even more enticing to Swedes who were tired of years of grinding poverty. By 1900 so many Swedes had emigrated that every sixth Swede lived in America. The outflux of Swedes had begun about 1840 and was inspired in part by a government edict which earlier in the century had divided the farmlands of Sweden into plots too small to sustain families.

Lund, my father's place of birth, is a historic area of Sweden. It is ten miles northeast of Malmo, the largest city in southern Sweden. It was founded a thousand years ago by the Danish King Canute the Great, and was the Roman Catholic capital of a region which stretched from Iceland to Finland. During that period it boasted a score of churches and half a dozen monasteries. Lund University was founded in the 1660's. Sweden conquered the province in 1679. Catholicism eventually gave way to Lutheranism, and in 1846 the first Swedish Lutheran Mission College was established. The arrival of the railroads in the 1860's brought industrial prosperity to the area. It is the site of a massive cathedral, begun in 1680, in the Romanesque style which is rare for that part of the world. Tourists marvel at its huge ornate, astronomical clock with intricate machinery that still plays daily at noon.

I can imagine Nils and his friend on the day they left

Lund taking a farewell look at the elaborate cathedral clock and wondering if they would ever see it again. But knowing young men as I do (being the mother of two sons), I'm sure the excitement of their plans for crossing the broad Atlantic Ocean far outweighed any pangs they felt at leaving their home and families.

We have no record of what ship the young men boarded, or from what port they departed. Perhaps they sailed on one of the three new ships acquired the year before by the Thingvalla Line (later to become the Scandinavian-American Line). The ships had steerage capacity for 600 emigrants. The Nordic Heritage Museum in Seattle has a replica of the cramped steerage quarters on such a ship, with its multiple narrow wooden bunks. At the time my father left Sweden, steerage conditions had improved considerably over the voyages that took place before 1868, when a bill was passed entitling steerage passengers to light, air, and food. One can only guess at the dreadful conditions which prompted such legislation, and the privations suffered by those desperate to escape oppression and poverty.

Even at the time my father made the voyage, sharing cramped quarters below decks with 600 persons (many of them no doubt suffering the misery of seasickness) must have been quite an ordeal. Although ship disasters were few and far between, they were frightening enough to discourage the faint-hearted. In 1904 the Norway, a ship bearing a load of Scandinavian emigrants, hit a reef off Scotland at full speed and sank rapidly, with the loss of 627 lives. It seems likely that the 168 who were rescued represented the first class passenger list, not those trapped in steerage. Nils and his friend may have known of similar disasters, but probably felt about them as most of us do about a plane crash. We know it would be horrifying, but are pretty sure it won't happen to us.

The young men were fortunate enough to arrive in Boston rather than New York, thereby escaping the mob scene which ensued when boatloads of weary travelers were processed at Ellis Island. The process of registration was simpler in Boston. Nils and his friend cleared the immigration hurdles without difficulty and changed their meager supply of Swedish money to American dollars. They were now entirely on their own, and neither of them spoke a word of English! My father had the equivalent of a high school education in Sweden, but English had not been on the curriculum.

As Nils and young Wiemer walked down the street in Boston they came upon a fruitstand. The colorful wares must have looked very appealing after the limited diet they had endured on board ship. Sign language was the order of the day. They pointed to a large stalk of bananas and handed the vendor a dollar bill. They hoped this would purchase at least one banana apiece, but to their surprise they were handed the entire stalk! They lugged it away, eating as they went. The first few bananas tasted wonderful, but finally they had reached their limit and they deposited the stalk on the sidewalk for the benefit of the next hungry person who came by. As long as he lived, my father had no further desire to eat a banana or anything that might contain bananas.

I have few details of my father's travels when he first

arrived in this country. The record does show that from Boston he went to Gerard, Illinois. Perhaps his companion had relatives there. He knew that if he was to realize his dream of becoming a doctor, he would have to work hard to pay for his education. In Gerard, along with many other Swedes, he found work in the mines. But while the others struggled with picks and shovels, he found another way to earn his living. They used donkey carts to transport the ore deep in the mines. My father rode the carts up and down the length of the mines selling insurance policies to miners. He was beginning to learn a little English, and he managed to memorize the contents of the insurance policies so that he could sell them successfully. He made enough money at this to get him started on his studies. Many years later I returned with him to Gerard to visit the family with which he had lived.

From Gerard we next find Nils in Denver, his brother Erik having settled near there. Erik probably had learned the tailoring trade from his father, for he worked as a tailor in this country. It must have been a touching scene when the two young brothers were reunited. Nils brought Erik heartwarming greetings from the loved ones in Sweden he missed so much, and Erik had many words of advice which could smooth the path for his newly arrived brother. Nils learned that in order to study medicine at the University of Colorado at Denver, he would have to learn not only the English language, but American history as well. He studied both subjects intensively and then was on his way toward a medical degree.

In those days it was not as complicated to become a physician as it is now, with the endless postgraduate courses and residencies that are required before today's M.D. can hang out his or her shingle. But even then, financing a medical education was no small feat. Nils worked in drugstores (they were open 24 hours a day then), and also as a night watchman on the streets of Denver. He carried his books and notes with him and studied whenever an opportunity presented itself, sometimes by the light of a gaslamp on a street corner.

He took his internship at St. Luke's Hospital in

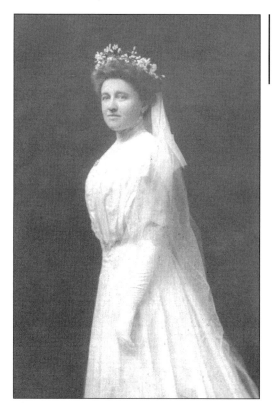

My mother, Katharine Adele Brown, on her wedding day.

Denver. At last the day came when he was fully qualified to practice medicine. The year was 1904. Can you imagine the joy that was felt by his family back in Lund when they received that first letter signed Nils August Johanson, M.D.? The news would have travelled up and down the street on which his family lived, perhaps inspiring yet another youngster to dream of America, the land of unlimited possibilities.

In the year after he got his medical degree he received an appointment to teach in the University's medical department, and was appointed to the medical staff of St. Anthony Hospital. The following year he received a staff appointment at the Jewish United Aid TB Sanatorium in Colorado. He began to contribute articles to newspapers and medical journals, including the Colorado Medical Times.

The young doctor had a great feeling of accomplishment after all his hard work. When he opened his first small office for surgical practice the income was slow in appearing. He had to sleep in his office as he couldn't afford to rent living quarters. Gradually he began to see more patients, however, and he felt comfortable enough in his new role to begin to enjoy some social life. Judging from his early photographs, Nils was a handsome young man who probably would have been considered quite a catch by the young women of Denver.

An attorney friend introduced him to Miss Katharine Adele Brown, a beautiful brunette. He promptly fell in love with her, and she with him.

Katharine's family background was quite different from that of the young Swedish immigrant. Her ancestors had come to America from Birmingham, England in 1636. She was descended from Major General Robert Sedgewick, who was appointed as the first military governor of Jamaica after the British captured it in 1653. Katharine's father was a prosperous wholesale grocer. He owned the J.S. Brown Mercantile Company, which had branches in Pueblo, Trinidad and Denver, Colorado.

The disparity in family backgrounds offered no impediment to the course of true love, however, and Katharine's parents welcomed the pleasant young doctor with the Swedish accent into their family. My mother was born on March 13, 1876, so she was thirty-one and Father was thirty-five when they were married. The couple was married in the home of the bride's parents in Denver, in 1907.

During the first year of their married life Katharine suffered from severe asthma which Nils believed was due to an allergy to some plant material in the Denver environment. He suggested that a change of climate might improve her health. Before long he closed his medical office in Denver, and the Johansons were en route to Tacoma, Washington. I believe this was toward the end of 1907. Although I don't doubt that my mother's asthma problem was very real, I think it is possible that the move westward was not entirely on that account. All of his life my father welcomed the challenge of new frontiers. He loved the great unexpected, and I feel sure he would have considered the settling of the far west as an enticing prospect. Be that as it may, my mother's asthma did clear up after the move.

In those days an interurban train ran between Tacoma and Seattle. Shortly after they were settled in Tacoma, Nils and Katharine decided to visit the growing metropolis of Seattle. Tacoma and Seattle were vying for the position as leading city of the Pacific Northwest. After seeing Seattle, Nils believed that it had a better chance to achieve this goal than did Tacoma. He and Katharine packed up their few belongings and moved to a residential hotel in Seattle. My father passed the Washington state medical examination in January, 1908, and opened his first Seattle office in Suite 405-6 of the Eitel Building, at the corner of Second Avenue and Pike Street, for the practice of surgery.

In Denver he had worked at large hospitals which were very advanced for that time. He found Seattle hospitals to be lacking in many respects. This was a period when the practice of medicine was undergoing some radical changes. Robert Koch's discovery of the tubercle bacillus in 1882 opened the door to recognition of the role that germs and bacteria played in human ills. 1891 marked the first use of rubber gloves in surgery to prevent the spread of bacteria. The invention of the x-ray had come in 1895, and the introduction of aspirin came in 1900. The 1902 discovery that human blood could be categorized into identifiable groups would radically change the course of surgery.

During the decade from 1880 to1890 the national death rate from abdominal and pelvic surgery dropped from 40 percent to less than 5 percent, due largely to the growing emphasis on hygienic surgical practices. In those days before the advent of antibiotics, if a surgical

patient developed a wound infection it would in all likelihood prove fatal. During his internship at St. Luke's
Hospital my father had learned that maintaining
scrupulously sterile surgical conditions was of lifesaving
importance.

He found to his dismay that Seattle hospitals were
not yet putting these new ideas into effect. As one
important medical milestone after another was reached,
it of course took some time for doctors and hospitals to
keep pace with such progress. Before long he realized
that if he was to practice surgery using the highest standards of sterile technique in which he had been trained,
he would have to establish his own hospital.

Chapter Two

From Summit to Swedish

As it entered the twentieth century Seattle was an energetic young community. In 1893 the Great Northern Railroad had connected the fledgling city with the rest of North America. The disastrous effects of the fire of 1889 had been overcome and businesses were beginning to thrive. Planked streets resounded with the sound of horses' hooves. By the time my father arrived in 1908 the first few automobiles had appeared on the streets of Seattle, but Duncan and Sons, the saddle and harnessmakers, still did a prosperous business. The tragic lesson of 1889 had been learned well and fire stations were strategically located. Passersby were wary when passing the stations, as at any moment the fire bell might clang, the station door would swing open, and a team of huge draft horses would charge out into the street, pulling the fire wagon with its tank of water and team of firefighters.

Plans were nearing completion for the Alaska-Yukon-Pacific Exposition to be held in Seattle in 1909.

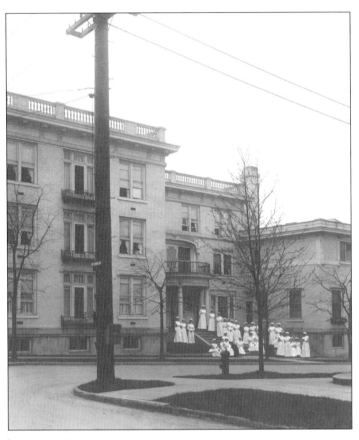

In the beginning,
Swedish Hospital

Its buildings began to take shape on a stretch of acreage north of Seattle to which the University of Washington had recently moved from its former downtown location. As newcomers to the community Nils and Katharine had begun to make friends. Because of his Swedish background, he was drawn toward others who had emigrated from his homeland. He became acquainted with a group of up and coming young business men who also had left Sweden to seek their fortunes in the new world. They had formed the Swedish Men's Business Club. He confided in his friends his desire to establish a hospital embodying all the standards of care he knew to be optimum, and they agreed to help him achieve this goal.

Nine of his friends each bought a $1,000 bond to raise money for my father's project, and lent their efforts to a fundraising drive. (Their investment later was repaid with interest.) They were P.A. Hallberg, J.A. Soderberg, John Kalberg, N.J. Nyquist, Emil Lovegren, Israel Nelson, Gustav A. Edelsvard, Godfrey Chealander and H.E. Turner.

Articles of Incorporation of Swedish Hospital were signed on June 13, 1908. The next two years saw a campaign to find a site and to raise funds. Concerts and banquets were held. The trustees set up a group to operate the Swedish Building at the Alaska-Yukon-Pacific Exposition in 1909 as a fund raiser, but unfortunately it made no money. Families and civic groups were encouraged to furnish a room in the proposed hospital. (Some families misunderstood that request, and offered household furniture they no longer needed.)

All of the Swedish community was behind this laudable effort of their countrymen, and $5,000 was raised through a bazaar at the Swedish Club. Various Swedish organizations sold tickets to name the queen of the bazaar, and the winning candidate represented the First Swedish Baptist Church. One reason for the strong community support was that Swedes living in the Pacific Northwest were grateful for the opportunities they had found in America. It was not enough that they contributed heavily to the area's development through activities such as logging and fishing. They wanted to do something concrete to express their appreciation, and the hospital gave them this opportunity.

On June 1, 1910, the founders signed a lease on a two-story apartment house at 1733 Belmont Avenue. Renovations were made, and in a few months Swedish Hospital accepted its first patients. My father realized that in order to achieve the standards of care to which he aspired, a skilled nursing staff would be necessary. Shortly after his new hospital opened its doors, he established the Swedish School of Nursing. By the time its first class of five young women graduated in 1913, the nursing school had moved with the hospital to another site.

While my father and his friends were raising money and making plans for the new hospital they believed the city required, another young Seattle doctor had been pursuing the same high purpose. He was Doctor Edmund M. Rininger. During the Alaskan gold rush Dr. Rininger had gone to Juneau to serve as a mines doctor, and in 1900 began his practice in Nome. In 1905 he moved his practice to Seattle, and apparently came to the same conclusion as my father, that if he wanted the kind of hospital he saw the need for he would have to establish it himself. Whether the two doctors were aware of each other's plans is not known, but I would think it was probable, in the small medical community.

Although Dr. Rininger began his plans for a hospital before my father arrived in Seattle, Swedish Hospital had already become a reality by the time Dr. Rininger's hospital neared completion. In 1905 he had purchased the home of C.J. Smith, (who was moving his residence to Harvard Avenue). He decided to buy the house next door to it for his own home, and make the Smith home, at 803 Summit, into a hospital. It was to be called Summit Hospital.

In 1911 Dr. Rininger spent three months in Europe visiting hospitals and searching for equipment. During his travels he met several young doctors whom he persuaded to come to Seattle to practice medicine in conjunction with the new Summit Hospital.

Meanwhile my father and his friends had encountered some problems. Their efforts had brought Swedish Hospital into being in a comparatively brief time frame, but shortly after the opening it became apparent that the building at 1733 Belmont was not adequate for their needs, because of space and layout limitations. Then too, there was the problem of the neighbors, who had nothing against the new hospital except that they wanted it located in someone else's neighborhood. The Board of Trustees decided that a larger site was a necessity. At this point fate stepped in.

Doctor Rininger was by now completing last minute details of the furnishings for his hospital. He must have had the same feelings of exhilaration and anticipation that my father and his friends experienced as their plans for Swedish Hospital reached fruition. Doctor Rininger had encountered more problems initially, however, than the Swedish group. He survived three lawsuits before a permit was issued for his hospital, but finally the contract for construction was signed early in March, 1912, and he moved his family from their residence which was on the site.

By the summer of 1912 the Summit Hospital was very close to completion. Doctor Rininger was an automobile enthusiast and on page 29 there is a picture of him seated as a passenger in the third privately-owned car in Seattle. On July 25, 1912, Doctor Rininger drove his automobile to Kent, Washington, to visit a patient and to inspect the hospital beds being manufactured there. On his way home his car was struck by the electric train which ran between Tacoma and Seattle and Doctor Rininger was killed, at the age of 42. He was said to be Seattle's first auto fatality.

His widow, Mrs. Eleanore Rininger, was of course devastated at the loss of her husband, and she was particularly saddened that he had not lived to see his hospital become a reality. When her husband's estate was being settled she was advised to sell the nearly complete hospital for use as an apartment house. She could not bring herself to do this, however. She wanted to see her husband's dream come true, and she saw a way this could be accomplished. She began negotiations with the

Board of Trustees of Swedish Hospital.

One story has it that in her effort to interest the Board in purchasing the completely equipped Summit Hospital Mrs. Rininger pointed out that the mono-grammed china already on hand bore the initials S.H., which could just as readily stand for Swedish Hospital. On December 9, 1912, the Board of Trustees authorized the purchase of Dr. Rininger's hospital for $90,723, plus an additional amount of $4,200 for hospital equipment.

My father had been the prime mover in seeing the need for Swedish Hospital and getting the ball rolling toward fulfilling that need. Once the hospital was estab-lished as a nonprofit corporation, further decisions were

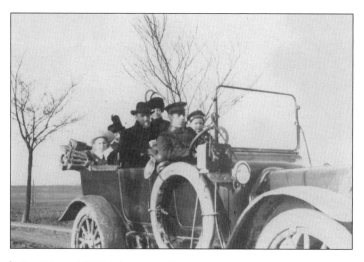

Dr. Edmund M. Rininger, seated behind driver of his automobile, one of the first in the Seattle area

made by its Board of Trustees, of which he was a member.

It was a most unusual Board -- a group of unselfish men whose desire to provide the very best hospital facilities possible was equaled only by their devoted friendship with one another. The original bylaws required that all Board members be of Swedish descent, so they shared that common bond. The trustees during the hospital's infancy were men whose training in various fields proved of invaluable aid in establishing the institution. They were determined to run the hospital on a business-like basis, taking advantage of the special background of each member.

There was P.A. Hallberg, who was a restaurant owner and served as culinary expert. Otto Roseleaf was a builder, H. E. Turner was a produce man, and Andrew Chilberg was a banker. Carl Wallin, Herman Peterson, John Isaacson, J.S. Soderberg, and C.S. Johnson all were respected businessmen. Doctor Johanson represented the medical profession. As the hospital progressed and improvements were made, the advice of these men saved many thousands of dollars which would have been required to obtain professional advice.

The new hospital was dedicated on March 16, 1913. It included a room designated as "The Rininger Memorial Library," containing Doctor Rininger's medical library, which had been presented by his widow. At the monthly meeting of board members on March 14, 1913, proceedings were interrupted when a nurse appeared with a small bundle containing the first baby born in the new hospital. The brand new son of Mr. and

Mrs. Magnus Johnson was made an honorary board member for life, and members took up a collection with which to purchase a silver cup for the infant.

In these days when hospital construction or remodeling involves millions of dollars, the $90,000 indebtedness which my father and fellow Board members incurred to purchase the new hospital in 1912 sounds rather minimal. But at that time it was a tremendous amount of money to borrow. An initial cash outlay of $27,000 was obtained through the sale of ten-year second mortgage hospital bonds. The Board's president, J.S. Soderberg made a substantial subscription toward the purchase.

Throughout the 40 years that my father supervised the Swedish Hospital's operation, he went to the bank many times to borrow large sums of money for improvements, and he was always able to get what he needed. I think the banks must have been impressed not only with the strong business background of Board members, but by my father's sincere desire to bring the very best in medical care to the growing Seattle area.

The new Swedish Hospital, on the corner of Summit and Columbia, had a bed capacity of 40. Its main entrance was on Summit. The hospital was a success from the very beginning. Just two years after its purchase the pattern of expansion began which has continued throughout the years, so that presently Swedish Medical Center occupies twenty blocks.

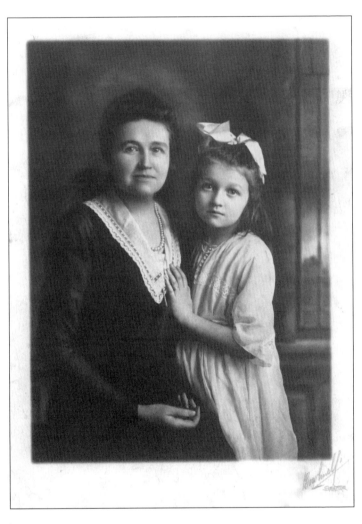

My mother and I

Chapter Three

Miss Kitty

It seems strange to me that even though my father had just founded a new hospital, I was born at home. Perhaps that was my mother's choice. I was born May 9, 1911, and named Katharine, after my mother. I guess that seemed like a pretty long name to tack on a tiny baby, so from the beginning I was called Kitty.

I was born at 2800 Broadway East (at Hamlin) on Capitol Hill in Seattle. My father had the house built in 1909. It's a historic Seattle house because it was designed in the Swiss chalet style by the prominent early day architectural firm of Cutter, Malmgren, who also designed the Seattle Golf Club and other well known Seattle buildings. It was a lovely house to grow up in. Elmer and I were married there. I've driven by the house in recent years and noted that subsequent owners have added on to the back of it, but it's been kept in very good condition. My parents continued to live there until the 1940's, when they sold it and moved to a house in Denny Park, on the north end of Lake Washington.

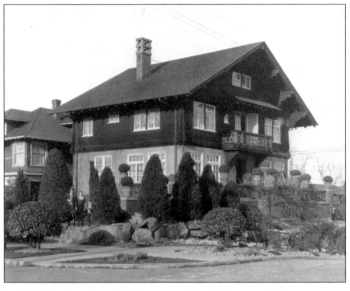

This is the house in which I grew up. It's still there, at 2800 Broadway East, in Seattle.

Being an only child has its privileges and its short-comings. I'm glad my two sons each had the advantage of growing up with a brother. They are very good friends and are closely associated in the family business. Sometimes an only child can be the recipient of a little too much loving attention, which was probably true in my case. I attended first grade at a public school and was enjoying it very much, but in playing with the other children I contracted scabies on my hands. This cleared up quickly, but my father's interest in maintaining sterile conditions apparently extended to the way he wanted his child cared for. He promptly took me out of public school and hired a private tutor for me. I didn't return to a classroom situation until I reached high school.

I'm sure Father thought he had my best interests at heart, but it was very hard on me to miss out on attending school during all those years. I used to watch my little friends walking by our house on their way to school and I really wanted to be one of them. I did have them as playmates after school, however, so it wasn't total isolation.

During the years I was growing up my father was extremely busy. He not only was a leading surgeon in Seattle, but also had the responsibility of running the hospital. Usually he was home for dinner, but our household had to be on a pretty flexible schedule as far as meals were concerned. We ate things like steaks or chops that could be cooked quickly after Father walked in the door. He quite often would be delayed by his surgical duties or a hospital meeting. After dinner he might allow himself the luxury of ten or fifteen minutes in which to sit down in the living room and read the paper, but then he would leave to make evening rounds of his surgical patients at the hospital. He could never go to bed at night unless he had made his rounds.

He made house calls at night also. Sometimes I would accompany him. One night he got a call after dinner that he was needed in Issaquah because of an accident of some sort, and I went along. We picked up a little boy who had been badly hurt and drove him in town to the hospital. My mother often accompanied my father on his calls, and welcomed these opportunities to spend some time with her busy husband.

My father made house calls on patients as far afield as Black Diamond or Enumclaw, but most of his calls

My father shared his love of riding with me.

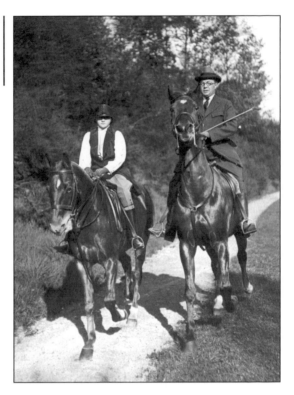

were in the Seattle area. This would have been around 1915 or 1920, and the roads weren't all that good, even in the city. They were unpaved, and many of the sidewalks were made of planks. Father had a huge spotlight on his car which could be tilted at any angle. I can picture him now, driving along a dirt road in the dark with house numbers barely visible, shining that big light up onto porches looking for the right number.

He was quite indulgent with me in most respects, and was not a strict disciplinarian. When you are an only child there probably is less need for corrective action. Parents are spared the inevitable squabbles among siblings that require refereeing. I never had any household responsibilities, as we always had help. I think that children should have some regular duties, no matter how affluent the household. Our sons had paper routes when they were boys, and I believe the experience was good for them--even if I did end up delivering the route myself sometimes in an emergency! My husband recalled that one morning I asked him to take the Cadillac to work and leave me the Ford. "Why?" he asked. I replied that because our son was ill I was going to have to deliver his Times route, and I wasn't about to do it in a Cadillac!

From my earliest recollections of our family life my father and I had a special affinity--we just enjoyed each other's company a great deal. When I was nine years old Father took up horseback riding as a sport, and this was something we did together. I had a cute little riding outfit, and we had our boots specially made, as you couldn't buy them at a store. We rode at the Olympic Riding Academy, which my father helped to found. It originally was on Lake Washington Boulevard near Madison, and I can remember the big old Park Department stable down there. Father and the other men helped establish trails through wooded areas. We had a path all the way along the boulevard. There was a big wide place in the Arboretum which we called the speedway, because a lot of horses could ride through there together. When Broadmoor was opened we used to ride in there a great deal.

That was in the early 1920's. The city began closing in on that area, so the Riding Academy founders got together and bought property out on Roosevelt Way, at about 110th I believe. We rode out there for years. The Academy is gone now, and when I tried to get some information about its exact former location none of the present-day riding people knew anything about it! But I have such wonderful memories of those days, riding along at my father's side, just enjoying being with him, loving the horses and the riding experience, and the great outdoors. We had four or five horses of our own. When the Olympic Riding Academy moved north, Father built a small stable right across the street from it where he kept our horses. One night our groom apparently fell asleep with a cigarette and burned down the stable, but luckily neither he nor the horses were hurt.

The wooded areas we enjoyed so much with the original Olympic Riding Academy were very near the Madison Park area where I now spend part of the year in my condominium. The woods of course are long gone-- the price of progress. It hardly seems like the same city that I knew as a child. One has to go pretty far afield now to find places where people still ride horses.

My parents had a very happy marriage, but there were some interests they just did not share, and riding was one of them. Getting on a horse was about the last thing on earth my mother would have thought of doing. She also refused absolutely to learn to drive a car. She was really a Victorian lady. She did beautiful needlework. I've seen some of the clothes she made for me as a baby and they were simply beautiful--lots of tiny tucks and lace. She enjoyed making our home an attractive and welcoming haven for my father that he could enjoy in the short periods between his many responsibilities. She came from a rather large family. Her mother died of cancer at age 36, when my mother was only five years old. Her father remarried, and had a total of ten children--I believe five by each wife. He died at age 72.

My mother's life revolved around Father's working hours but she learned to cope very well with this, and I think was happy in her own routine. She played bridge and was an active member of a Children's Orthopedic guild--these were just getting started then. I joined one myself after I was married.

Father belonged to the Seattle Golf Club, but when he became so interested in riding horseback he practically gave up golf. My parents' social life together consisted mostly of small dinner parties at our home or the homes of friends, and occasionally the three of us would go out to dinner together. When radio was invented in the 1920's, that provided a big interest for most families of that day, ours included.

Father used to take me to his office sometimes, which for many years was downtown on 4th Avenue. The nurses always made a big fuss over me. On Sunday mornings when we'd go horseback riding he would always have to make his rounds, so we'd go to the hospital first, and I'd sit in the lobby and visit with the admitting staff.

Even though I missed out on attending school with my chums, we did have fun together as playmates. We enjoyed riding our bicycles together. I had a lot of pets, too. At one time we had a little bulldog, a Pomeranian and three hunting dogs (a pointer and two English setters). Hunting and fishing were both avid interests of my father. He loved pheasant and duck hunting. He belonged to a duck club, and used to go hunting up near Bellingham with a Mr. Purdy, who was a pioneer settler up there.

John Soderberg has been on the Board for many years, as was his father. John Soderberg, Senior, was one of the founders, and often came to the financial aid of the hospital during the early years. His original trade was as a stonemason, although he later had many interests and was very successful. He built a house of granite on Broadway East in 1910, right across from our house. Back in 1911, at about the same time I was born, the Soderbergs across the street welcomed a new little son, John, Jr., (also born at home). Because I didn't attend public school as a child, I didn't have much contact with John at that time. However, we have been friends through the years because he and Elmer were fellow Swedish Hospital board members for so long. John's father was on the board until his death in 1935, and John has been a board member since 1942.

A major interest of our family was our vacation home on Hood Canal, which my parents bought when I was about eight years old--but more about that later.

Holidays were of course exciting times as a child. At Thanksgiving and Christmas we quite often got together with my father's family. In addition to his brother Erik, two of Father's sisters also lived in Seattle. Rika's husband, Elof Swenson, worked in inventory control at Swedish Hospital, and Anna's husband, Max Schertle, was a professor of German at the University of Washington. Erik Johanson's son, Perry, and I shared the same birthday, although he was a year older than me.

40

Perry's older brother was Nels.

Father and his brother and sisters enjoyed talking about their early years together in Sweden. He loved his parents very much, and I'm sure he missed having the opportunity to see them. Now that Elmer and I are blessed with our children, grandchildren and even great grandchildren, the special occasions when we all are able to get together for family celebrations are so enjoyable for us. I'm sorry that my father did not have the opportunity to share his life with his parents as they grew older. He did return to Lund from time to time to visit them, however. My cousin, Signe Ahlbin, who lived in Stockholm, was the daughter of Father's brother, Gustaf. She remembered my father's visits to Sweden when she was a youngster. She was told that my father had a portrait of his mother in Seattle which fell to the floor. He took this as an omen, apparently, and made a visit to Sweden to see his parents. Later that year his mother died. His father lived to the age of 93.

Not all of my father's friends were Swedes, but he had an understandable affection for and appreciation of those with Swedish blood. This seems pretty evident from the clause he included in the original Swedish Hospital bylaws requiring that all Board members be of Swedish descent. My father claimed there was no chauvinism involved here -- it was just that Swedes were such good business men! That requirement was removed from the bylaws in 1970, but because some of the original members had sons or grandsons who are now on the Board, there still is enough Swedish blood there to keep things on a very business-like basis!

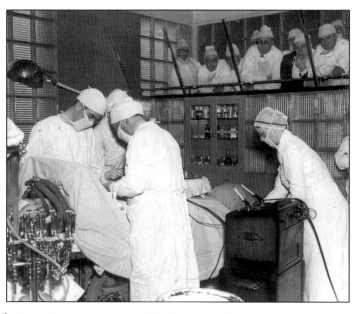

An early day surgery at Swedish Hospital, with my father in the foreground. Note the keenly interested spectators.

Chapter Four

A Staff of Strength

M y father believed that providing the hospital with
a highly qualified staff was at least as important
a consideration as building the facilities to care for
patients. There were eight or ten doctors on the active
staff of the new hospital. Among them were several who
had been brought to Seattle by Doctor Rininger. On the
trip he made to Europe to get ideas for his hospital he
met Doctor Carl Leede, an American who was Research
Assistant at the Eppendorf Hospital in Hamburg,
Germany. He was very impressed with Doctor Leede,
and through subsequent correspondence it was agreed
that the young physician would come to Seattle as a staff
member at Doctor Rininger's hospital in September,
1912. He was engaged to a German girl. They had just
arrived at his mother's house in Washington, D.C. in
July, 1912, when they learned of Doctor Rininger's
untimely death.

Doctor Leede decided to go ahead with his plans to
practice in Seattle, and he and his fiancee were married

in Mrs. Rininger's home, on the present Swedish Hospital site. He became a staff member at Swedish Hospital, and remained on the staff until his retirement in 1949. His three children were born at Swedish Hospital. One daughter was named Eleanore, after Mrs. Rininger. His son, Doctor William Leede, also was on the Swedish staff for many years.

At the time of his arrival in Seattle Doctor Leede was the only doctor in this area who specialized in internal medicine. The field of diagnosis was one in which most doctors had little or no training, and it had therefore become commonplace to perform many exploratory operations. Swedish Hospital played a prominent part in eliminating this practice by providing excellent training in the field of diagnosis, so that the field of internal medicine became firmly established.

Doctor Otis Floyd Lamson, who had completed advanced surgical training with the Mayo brothers in Rochester, Minnesota, was another young doctor who was persuaded to come to Seattle by Doctor Rininger. Doctor Lamson proved to be a strong addition to the Swedish Hospital staff and had a long and distinguished medical career in Seattle. When he was interviewed during the 1950's he recalled that soon after its beginnings, Swedish emerged as a leading hospital because of the modern and progressive methods instituted by my father. "Other hospitals which have been well established in Seattle at one time or another," said Doctor Lamson, "have fallen behind in size and scope because their leadership was not as progressive as that of Swedish."

The hospital was under the direct management of my

father from the beginning, and the high standards he set are responsible to a large degree for the splendid reputation which Swedish Hospital maintains today. He required that every person connected with the hospital in any capacity be well qualified and of good character. His tremendous enthusiasm inspired the high degree of efficiency which he required of staff members. He visited hospitals in this country and in Europe in his search for modern methods of treatment and the newest of equipment. Swedish pioneered in the use of much equipment which is standard to all hospitals today.

When blood transfusions were almost unheard of, Doctor William Speidel, who had received special training from the inventor of this technique, gave successful transfusions at Swedish. In those days it was necessary to anesthetize both donor and receiver, making an incision in the wrist of each and joining the veins directly. Doctor Speidel's son, William, wrote some popular books about early-day Seattle, and was the founder of the Seattle Underground Tours.

Another member of that early day staff at Swedish was Doctor S. Maimon Samuels, who had been trained in performing "bloodless" tonsillectomies under local anesthesia. This was a technique new to the practice of surgery, and some of the first such operations were performed at Swedish Hospital by Dr. Samuels. When interviewed in the 1950's he recalled that Swedish was the first hospital in this area to allow patients a menu choice. It was recognized that anything which helps the patient feel more content will speed his recovery. A system was set up whereby the patient was given a diversified menu from which to select his or her meals. This of course is common practice in today's hospitals, but was a welcome innovation then.

Swedish Hospital pioneered in many areas, such as providing the first all-glass surgery in the United States. Because of its reputation for being in the forefront of hospital design and equipment Swedish is of great interest to hospital administrators throughout the country, and frequent requests for information on the operation of various departments are received.

My father's desire to staff the Swedish Hospital with only the best qualified physicians had an impact on the practice of medicine in the Pacific Northwest which continues to this day. Although most of the staff members my father hired are no longer living, there is one among them who still plays a leading role in the area of medical research. He is Doctor William B. Hutchinson, well known for having established the Fred Hutchinson Cancer Research Center, and presently serving as president and director of the Pacific Northwest Research Foundation. Doctor Hutchinson's younger brother was Fred Hutchinson, prominent sports figure in baseball, whose life was cut short by cancer at age 43.

When asked about his first contact with my father, Doctor Hutchinson replied: "He changed my whole professional career. My father was a physician in the Rainier Beach area. I had received excellent training at Johns Hopkins in Baltimore, but I loved the Pacific Northwest, and wanted to take up my practice of surgery here. I returned from the east in January, 1940, and became a staff member at Providence Hospital.

"Because my father took his patients to Providence Hospital, I knew a lot of men on the staff and it was a natural place for me to work. But my eastern training had been rather formal, and it did not quite agree with some of the methods I was forced to use there. Probably the most distressing was the trouble I had in scheduling my cases and knowing when I was going to operate, because older men on the staff would be given preference. After I had scheduled a case four or five days in advance, it suddenly would be moved to make way for an older doctor's patient. This became a source of great anxiety for me.

"One day I was doing some surgery at Harborview, the county hospital, with Doctor Homer Dudley. He was a good friend, and I told him I was having so much trouble that I had to do one of two things: Either get a different place to work, or go back to Baltimore. I had received several good offers to practice there with well established surgeons but I hated to leave Seattle.

"Doctor Dudley said, 'Well, this morning I have a meeting scheduled with Doctor Nils Johanson, the head of Swedish Hospital. Would you mind if I asked him whether he'd be interested in talking to you?' Of course I said, 'Not at all.'

"Later that morning I got a call from Doctor Johanson, asking if I could have lunch with him that day, which I did. He was very cordial, and asked me if I would be interested in working at Swedish Hospital. I told him that I had only an occasional patient, but would be tickled to death to work at Swedish. He promptly took me upstairs and introduced me to Miss Tysdale, superintendent of the nursing staff in the operating room. He told her he was anxious to have me work at Swedish and asked her to be sure I had everything I needed in the way of instruments. He said to her, 'Now if there's anything you don't have that Doctor Hutchinson needs, I want to know about it.'

"I was amazed, because for the first time in the year that I had been back in Seattle I had been asked what equipment I would like to work with. From that time on I worked chiefly at Swedish, and it was always a great pleasure to work there. Doctor Johanson looked after me in great style.

"Two or three years after I joined the staff at Swedish, Doctor Johanson told me he was moving his office into the hospital and asked if I would like to take over the office he was leaving, which I did. They were small, one-story offices, at 1310 Madison. I was very fond of Doctor Johanson. He was a man of great foresight. He was able to detect those areas of medicine which showed great promise. I think the best evidence of that was his interest in the treatment of cancer by X-ray. When he established the Tumor Institute at Swedish Hospital in 1932 he was way ahead of his time.

"Some of his ideas were so advanced that I'm sure he must have had trouble from time to time in persuading the Board to go along with him. But he had great perseverance, and with his knowledge of medicine and his uncanny foresight, he was able to get his ideas acted upon favorably. When he needed financial support for new projects, I think the bankers recognized his great integrity and wanted to deal with him because he was very successful.

"Doctor Johanson travelled frequently, both here and abroad, to obtain new ideas. This really was a necessity, as medicine here was quite primitive, and there were exciting changes going on elsewhere. He was always looking for the opportunity to bring in people who were outstanding in their field. When he learned of the progress in radiation therapy for the treatment of cancer, he brought in Doctors Simeon Cantril and Franz Buschke, both of very high reputation in this new field. This just made the Tumor Institute.

"Under his direction the hospital grew rapidly, and particularly after World War II it grew by leaps and bounds. The progress which it continues to make is a tribute to the strong foundation it received under Doctor Johanson's leadership."

In the above account by Doctor Hutchinson, I learned of one more instance where an action of my father enriched the practice of medicine for others and elevated the status of the hospital he loved. What a loss it would have been to Seattle if Bill Hutchinson had followed his early impulse to return to Baltimore to practice surgery. Not only did he become a valued staff member at Swedish, but both of the research facilities with which his name has become synonymous have achieved major recognition and have added greatly to the body of medical knowledge.

One thing that Doctor Hutchinson mentioned was quite typical of my father. On the morning Father learned from Doctor Dudley that Bill Hutchinson was unhappy at Providence, he did not make a note to get in touch with him sometime later. He invited him to lunch that day, and added him to the staff at once. He was capable of making intuitive decisions without delay, and he was not a procrastinator. Another point demonstrated in Doctor Hutchinson's account was my father's insistence that the young doctor be provided with everything he needed to perform his surgeries under optimum conditions. He wanted the hospital to offer a strong support system to staff members.

Chapter Five

With Loving Care and Healing Hands

"For your professional care, dedication and hard work each of you deserves special recognition today and every day. We depend on you."

These words of praise appeared in a two-page newspaper ad with which the Swedish Medical Center honored its nursing staff a few years ago on National Nurses' Day. The names of all nurses on the hospital staff were included in the ad.

This grateful recognition of the important role which nurses have played in the success of Swedish Hospital dates back to the day the hospital opened its doors in 1910. My father always was aware of the importance of skilled nursing care, which is the reason he founded a school of nursing within the same year the hospital was established.

To realize the important role the nurse played in the early days of the hospital, you have to consider the state of medical practice in those days. Surgery was of a very primary nature. There were few drugs and of course none of the antibiotics which play such an important role today. X-ray had just been discovered a few years before, and it was to be many decades before the complex diagnostic tools we now depend upon would evolve. If you were very ill the hospital could provide rest, quiet and physical care to help you regain your health. Nursing care was a major part of what the early-day hospital had to offer.

The many scientific discoveries which have altered the practice of medicine since the founding of Swedish Hospital have also affected the educational requirements for skilled nursing. Early day nurses carried bedpans, bathed patients, took temperatures, served the meals, and administered what medicines were available. The quotient of tender loving care which they offered was a major factor in the patient's recovery and this is equally true of today's nurse. In addition, however, today's hospital nurse must deal with a great deal of technology.

If a cancer patient is receiving drugs through four separate chemotherapy pumps, the attending nurse must understand how those pumps work. She also should know that the drugs used to deliver the chemotherapy can be absorbed through her skin and could alter her own body chemistry if she does not wear protective gloves. She must observe necessary precautions to avoid excessive exposure when delivering radiation therapy.

With the emergence of Swedish Hospital as a neonatal center, nurses need to know how to handle and care for a premature infant which may weigh less than two pounds. There are 4,000 babies born each year at Swedish. At the time the hospital was founded, general surgeons also delivered babies on occasion, since there were not as many specialists in obstetrics in those days. The first baby born at the original Swedish Hospital, in 1910, was delivered by my father. He also transported the expectant mother from her home on Queen Anne to the hospital, over some very bumpy roads.

Whenever newly devised medical equipment appears on the scene, nurses must be educated to deal with it. In recent years passersby have noticed that a large trailer is parked in the courtyard of Swedish Hospital Medical Center several times a week. It contains the equipment used for lithotripsy, the process in which kidney stones are disintegrated by a laser beam, without subjecting the patient to surgery. The process is relatively painless, but because of its newness it probably causes some concern in the patient. The presence of a skilled nurse who can explain the steps as the work proceeds is of great comfort to the patient. Incidentally, the lithotripsy equipment is housed in the trailer because it is shared with several other hospitals in order to minimize the cost of the treatment. Providing quality care at the lowest possible cost has always been a concern at Swedish.

During my father's lifetime the term hospice was not commonly used in the medical community, but now it is of great importance. Hospitals formerly placed major emphasis on the curing of patients. Those who could not be cured and went home to die were no longer considered the hospital's responsibility. In my father's time these patients would be attended by individual physicians, and many of the house calls he made were to those in the final stages of illness.

Eventually house calls became an impractical way of delivering medical care for the most part. Patients who were chronically ill or in the final stages of an illness and unable to get to the doctor's office did not receive the attention they should have. Those who served as their caretakers also were under considerable stress in caring for these invalids.

In recent years hospitals have recognized this gap in medical care, and thus the development of the hospice concept. In 1985 Swedish Hospital began its Sustaining Care program, a home health and hospice agency. The program was founded by Doctor Robert Mack, a respected vascular surgeon who had served as Swedish Hospital's Chief of Staff and headed many hospital committees. At the age of 49, Doctor Mack was diagnosed with cancer of the lung. He waged a valiant battle against this disease but it eventually took his life. Before he died, however, he had the satisfaction of seeing his dream fulfilled that Swedish would offer a program of care for terminally and chronically ill patients, providing continuity of care between hospital and home and attending physician.

Nurses are the backbone of Sustaining Care. They are on call 24 hours a day, 7 days a week. They need to be flexible, independent, and very skilled at assessing the patient's needs. Although 75% of the hospice patients die at home, it is up to the nurse to decide whether at some point the patient's welfare calls for a return to the hospital. The Sustaining Care nurses also work closely with the program's chaplain and must be aware of when his services would be most appreciated by the patient and the family.

Sustaining Care nurses usually have experienced the loss of loved ones themselves and have come to terms with their own mortality, at least to a certain degree. Their nature is to feel rewarded in offering loving care not only to the patient but to the caregiver, who often is greatly in need of the strong support system which Sustaining Care offers. Volunteers have also contributed greatly to this program.

Early records indicate my father's strong interest not only in providing the hospital's student nurses with training curriculum which would serve them well in their chosen profession, but also in offering them comfortable living conditions. Board minutes show that the young women were provided with an area in which to play tennis, and at one time the Hospital Board rented a summer cabin in West Seattle for their enjoyment during warm weather. Graduating nurses always were treated to a large family picnic by the hospital. For many years this outing was held at Hood Canal, and my family and I have participated in many of them. I remember the picnics as very happy occasions.

In a day when women's capabilities were not always recognized, my father showed a particular skill in hiring women to fill administrative positions, and also in giving them credit for the work they accomplished. He hired Herina Eklind, a registered nurse (also of Swedish descent!) in 1924 and in 1930 she became Director of Nurses. In 1946 she became Superintendent of the hospital, a position she occupied with great skill for many years. When a beautiful new nurses' home was built by Swedish in 1946 in response to my father's desire to provide comfortable and attractive quarters for the student nurses, the Board of Trustees recognized Miss Eklind's great contribution to Swedish by naming the building Eklind Hall.

The nursing school at Swedish eventually was combined with training at the University of Washington, and is no longer based at the hospital. Student nurses from nearby universities and community colleges are rotated through the hospital as a part of their training. I think my father would particularly approve of a later step which was taken to improve the skilled nursing care available to patients at Swedish. The hospital's Nursing Institute is an educational program which provides employees with training in every service, including surgery, obstetrics, critical care, dialysis, acute care, transplantation, and cardiac. The program enables someone already trained as a Licensed Practical Nurse to obtain an Associate Degree and become an RN.

In an affiliation with Seattle Pacific University, Swedish Hospital pays the tuition for RN's with an Associate Degree who wish to devote an additional two years to the Baccalaureate program, which greatly increases their opportunity to advance in administrative positions. In return for the quarters of tuition they receive, these students agree to work an equal number of quarters for the hospital, and the likelihood is great that many of them will spend many years in positions of responsibility on the hospital's staff. Ninety percent of the head nurses at Swedish have a Baccalaureate or

Master's Degree. This tuition-paid program is quite in keeping with my father's philosophy that skilled nurses were the heart of the hospital and deserved every advantage the hospital could offer them.

That Swedish Hospital is looked upon by nurses as an outstanding employer is borne out by the number of nurses who have worked there for thirty or forty years before retiring. The strong family feeling among staff members continues into retirement, and there are several get-togethers during the year arranged by those who formerly worked at Swedish. Among these are an annual picnic and a Christmas party. There is also a yearly luncheon for retired nurses which is sponsored by the medical center.

Chapter Six

Medical Education – A Lifelong Process

According to early records, my father seemed to have a gift for attracting the most skilled physicians to his hospital staff. He recognized early on, however, that the hospital he founded would have to share responsibility for providing physicians with the training and experience they needed. In 1920, he set up an internship program, and served as an instructor in surgery himself.

The outstanding physicians on that early-day staff, including Doctors Leede, Samuels, Lamson, and others, all contributed their expertise to the task of providing needed training for the young doctors who chose to intern at Swedish. Doctor Edwin Chase was one of those interns and he remembers that the surgical procedures he learned under my father's tutelage placed heavy emphasis on sterile technique. 'We scrubbed and scrubbed and scrubbed," he said, "and we were very, very careful...You were taught to get into a rhythm and get everything working well as a team, to shorten the operating time."

Until the arrival of antibiotics, infection could easily cause the patient's death even if the surgery itself had repaired the physical defect. My father's main reason for wanting his own hospital was to institute the standards of scrupulous sterile technique in which he had been trained. It is not surprising to me, therefore, that the training he offered his interns would heavily emphasize the need for strict cleanliness. In the book "Saddlebags and Scanners," a history of medical practice in the state of Washington (co-authored by Doctor James Haviland, a long time member of the Swedish medical staff) a discussion of Seattle's early-day hospitals included this statement: "...Swedish soon emerged as a leading hospital, due largely to the modern methods instituted by Dr. Johanson."

In 1937 a young doctor came to Swedish Hospital as an intern who was later to gain international recognition for his impact on the specialty of orthopedics. He was just out of Columbia University Medical School and had opportunities for internship in many places, including staying at Columbia, but he decided to accompany a friend who was interning at Swedish. And by just that chance decision, Seattle was to gain the great professional skill of Doctor Ernest Burgess. He became a pioneer in hip replacement surgery and was one of the first surgeons in the nation given permission to do this intricate operation. There followed a procession of visiting surgeons desirous of learning the hip replacement procedure from Doctor Burgess. Under the auspices of Swedish Hospital he trained more than two hundred surgeons from throughout the country in this procedure. He and his office colleagues have by now performed more than three thousand hip replacements, in addition to the replacement of other joints which also became established procedures.

In recent years Dr. Burgess has become known as one of the inventors of the "Seattle foot," a widely respected innovation in the field of prosthetic devices. In his office guest book one finds names of amputee patients from throughout the world who have received the benefit of his skill in the design and application of prostheses. He has set up a nonprofit organization, the Prosthetics Research Foundation, to provide prostheses to patients in need, and maintains offices and clinics in far-flung countries to pursue this worthwhile endeavor.

Ernest Burgess became a good friend of my father's during his internship, and has maintained friendly ties with my family throughout the years. He recalls with affection his year of internship at Swedish and has agreed to share his recollections of my father in these pages:

"I met Doctor Johanson two or three days after registering at the hospital," said Doctor Burgess. "He was quite a remarkable man, even at our first meeting. He was rather a short gentleman, stood very upright, and looked and acted in a professorial manner. He was friendly, but it was obvious from the start that he was a man who knew what he wanted to do. He was very definite and precise in his statements.

"He welcomed us, told us he was looking forward to

having a wonderful time with us in training. Our year of internship included three-month periods of rotation at Children's Orthopedic (which was then on Queen Anne), at Firlands Sanatorium, and at Seattle General Hospital. Dr. Johanson was responsible for the work we did at these other hospitals, as well as for our stint at Swedish.

"Dr. Johanson usually did three or four cases a day, and was an extremely skilled surgeon. I remember the first case in which I participated. It was a pelvic operation on a woman. As the operation was about to get started I noticed there was no anesthesiologist present. Lo and behold, Dr. Johanson gave his own spinal anesthesia to this lady. I thought that was quite unusual, but it turned out to be his regular practice. I had been an observer in top medical centers in New York, and had seen fine anesthesiologists at work there. I therefore recognized that Dr. Johanson was very, very skilled at administering spinal anesthesia.

"I don't think that operation took him 45 minutes. He didn't waste a movement. Everything was exactly like a skilled machine. I was very impressed that this man really knew what he was doing. When he came to the end of that case he said, 'All right, doctor, you go ahead and sew up this patient, and I'll get ready for the next patient.'

"Well, I thought, my golly, can I do this right? But I'd had some practice and I sewed up the skin. He popped in and out of the room to see that it was going all right, and it did.

"I believe there were six or eight interns in our group

that year. Dr. Johanson was determined that his interns were going to leave there knowing something about how to do surgery. Some of us would be going directly into general practice, and at that time many general practitioners did quite a bit of surgery — at least the simpler operations, such as appendectomies and tonsillectomies.

"As director of the hospital, Doctor Johanson was in the position of having to see that doctors didn't do surgery they weren't qualified to do. There were some hospitals, in those days, where if you came in and you were a doctor, you could do just about any surgery. There was not the close follow-up that there is now. It was a different situation at Swedish, however. Doctor Johanson was tactful about it, but in his hospital, doctors were not allowed to do surgery that did not correspond with their training. Swedish Hospital has always had very good patient control. That's why they've been able to maintain such an excellent staff.

"There weren't so many surgical specialists in those days. General surgeons did everything. Doctor Johanson would operate on the spine, did neurological surgery, he'd operate on stomachs, and was especially competent in tumor surgery. He'd do maxillofacial surgery, and all types of abdominal surgery. He was up here in a corner of the country with no medical school and no formal medical education going on except for what the doctors did locally. You'd have to go out of the city to get much in the way of postgraduate training. And yet here was a surgeon who was a very skilled, up-to-date, highly professional man. He could have worked anywhere in the world. And to combine that with keeping an eye on the entire operation of the hospital meant that he was a pretty busy fellow. He loved the hospital, you could just tell. He was very forward looking. He made Swedish a cancer center very early, one of the first such centers west of Chicago. He was way ahead of his time.

"I learned a lot from Doctor Johanson about surgery, and also about patient management. He was a natural teacher, but if he wasn't confident in what you could do, he wouldn't let you do anything. You just assisted. He was a fast surgeon. In those days we didn't have much in the way of antibiotics, and blood transfusions were direct, from donor to patient, so there was no extra time. Surgeons had to be very skillful.

"He was interested in all of his interns personally. I think Doctor Johanson took a special interest in me because he knew of my keen interest in surgery. I came from a family of physicians, and while still in high school had the opportunity to be an observer during many operations. He was very friendly with me. I was invited to dinner at his house several times, and while there I couldn't help noticing that he had a very pretty daughter. Kitty and I became good friends, and went out together socially. Over the years I have valued my friendship with Kitty and her husband, Elmer Nordstrom.

"Doctor Johanson knew of my interest in orthopedic surgery, and he introduced me to the outstanding orthopedic surgeons on his staff at Swedish. One of these was Doctor Roger Anderson. Doctor Johanson recommended to Doctor Anderson, who was a good friend of his, that after I had completed further training in orthopedics I would be a good man to work with him. When I completed my residency in New York I did join forces with Doctor Anderson, and became affiliated with Swedish Hospital. I was away in the war for a few years, and when I came back I immediately, reestablished myself at Swedish.

"I owe a debt of gratitude to Doctor Johanson, not only for the interest he took and the excellent training he offered, but for the fact that I met my wife, the former Ruth Anderson, through him. Ruth came down from Alaska to be Doctor Johanson's patient, and while she was in the hospital we got acquainted. We've been married for fifty-seven years now, so it looks like it's going to last!

"One of Doctor Johanson's qualities was that he was a no-nonsense fellow. He could be reserved and sometimes stern, but he also had a great deal of warmth. His life was centered around medicine, and Swedish Hospital was his life. He wanted it to be the best, and he succeeded. The amazing degree to which that success has continued beyond his lifetime is a great tribute to him."

Dr. Burgess's remarks demonstrated that once again my father had exerted a positive influence toward the betterment of medical practice in this town. By encouraging the association with Dr. Roger Anderson he saw to it that a very gifted young intern received the right opportunity to further his career in orthopedic surgery.

At the time Dr. Burgess interned, Swedish did not

have a residency program. Eventually it did develop advanced study programs which included two to three, or even five more years of training beyond internship. It was one of the early hospitals in Seattle to provide such training, and did so even before the University of Washington Medical School came on the scene in 1948.

Now that internships have been largely done away with in favor of resident programs, Swedish continues to offer training by a distinguished staff. It currently includes 52 resident physicians in its program, which is under the direction of Doctor John Wright, Director of Medical Education. The residency program was strengthened at the time of the merger of Seattle General, Doctors Hospital and Swedish Hospital, since Doctors also offered residencies, and Seattle General previously had. One particular strength which was gained with the merger was the addition of a residency program in Family Practice, which was started at Doctors Hospital under the direction of Doctor Frank Scardapane, who now heads the program for Swedish Hospital Medical Center. There are eighteen resident physicians in that program.

My father believed that a teaching hospital offered advantages not only to the physicians in training, but to those doctors who offered their knowledge in serving as teachers. He felt it was a challenge to all of his staff to deal with the questions and interests of these budding young doctors. The teaching program also helped him attract skilled physicians to his medical staff who had a particular interest in medical education.

In 1976 most states mandated that all physicians

would be required to show evidence they had taken a certain number of hours of additional training to update their skills in order to be re-licensed regularly. As a result, Swedish Medical Center offers a continuing variety of conferences and symposia in this program of keeping doctors' skills current.

In the early years of Swedish it was a comparatively simple matter to keep tabs on the medical staff to make sure that high standards of care were being met. This is a much more complicated matter now that the medical center has achieved such a dramatic growth. A very strict protocol is followed now in the review of charts, and if questionable care is indicated, the attending physician can be called to account by a committee which is responsible for quality control. Such supervision is essential if Swedish is to maintain its position of leadership in providing the highest quality of medical care combined with a diligent effort at cost control.

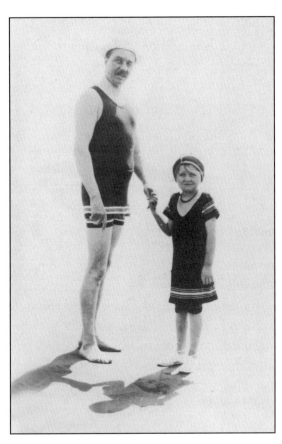

*Nils and daughter Kitty are ready
for a swim in Hood Canal.*

Chapter Seven

Hood Canal

I n about 1909 P. A. Hallberg, who came from
Sweden and operated a restaurant in Seattle, bought
a mile of waterfront property near Alderbrook on Hood
Canal. He divided it into 100 ft. waterfront lots and sold
them to several of his friends, including Carl Wallin,
John Nordstrom, and Otto Roseleaf. Some years later
one of the waterfront lots came up for re-sale and my
father bought it. I was eight when we first went to Hood
Canal. In those early years of the automobile it was an
all-day trip to get to Hood Canal, through Tacoma,
Olympia and Shelton. I suppose our top speed was 20
MPH. My mother and I would stay there for the entire
summer, with Father coming up for weekends.

During the first few years we lived in tents pitched
on a wooden platform, as did the other families who had
property there. Although it was camping out, it was not
quite as primitive as you might think. True, the cooking
was done on a camp stove, but it was done by our cook,
who came right along with us for the summer and had

her own tent.

Of course for the children, the slight inconveniences did not detract from the wonderful summer of fun on the saltwater beach. When it rained we would gather in a big stone house which all the families had the use of. We would also congregate there in the evenings after dinner. There was a windup Victrola which we all enjoyed, and the kids would play games.

There was a wonderful group of children to play with, including three boys and two girls in the Nordstrom family. The Nordstrom property was just a few lots down from ours. Lloyd, the youngest Nordstrom boy, was my special friend as he was my age. We had a lot of fun playing on the beach, and when we were teen-agers we once swam across Hood Canal together. The protected waters of the Canal are much warmer than most of the saltwater beaches in Washington, but as I recall, the water did get a little chilly before we made it across the Canal that day. We were accompanied by several boats so it really wasn't dangerous, and anyway, I float like a cork. After I was married I once swam across the widest part of the canal, with Elmer supervising from the rowboat.

During those summers I was allowed to bring a playmate along from the neighborhood. We did a lot of swimming in the canal, clam digging, and hiking through nearby woods. Sometimes we picked black-berries nearby. At night we often had a big bonfire and roasted wieners and marshmallows on sticks. It was a wonderful way to spend our summers.

At that time John Nordstrom and Carl Wallin were

partners in a small shoe store in Seattle, and they arranged their summer schedule so that each partner took an alternate week off to spend at Hood Canal. My father was able to come up only on weekends, although occasionally he would take a little vacation time to spend there also. I used to look forward to his arrival on Friday evening, and it was great to have him there all weekend. My mother enjoyed these times when she did not have to share her husband with the hospital rounds and house calls, which were such a part of his life when he was in the city.

We never knew what time Father would arrive on Friday night, but when I heard his car in the drive I'd run to give him a hug. On several occasions he drove up the driveway only to find a message waiting for him about an emergency. He'd have to turn right around, after that long drive, and go back to the city. While he was at the Canal he was always ministering to people who needed a doctor. Every Fourth of July it seemed there was a steady procession of burnt hands. One time he set a broken arm in the front yard. Elmer Nordstrom was a teen-ager then, and he held the top of the arm, Father held the bottom, and they applied a splint.

My father seldom took a lengthy vacation, but when I was about nine he had a minor heart problem and took a month off. We went to Delmar, California, and I remember the wonderful ocean beach there. By the end of the month Father was really chafing at the bit to get back to work.

Even in the country he never seemed to get the hang of just taking life easy. He always had many projects going. He was raising chinchilla rabbits, but they escaped and raided the neighbors' vegetable gardens, so he gave up on that and began raising mink. The idea was to sell the pelts to the European market. He had about 100 mink, which were doing nicely. A caretaker took care of them when we weren't there. One night some men tied up the caretaker, poisoned his dog, and stole all the mink. There was some evidence pointing to a local furrier, but nothing could be proved. That ended the Johanson mink ranch, and my father went on to other hobbies. We kept horses up there, and Father built some trout ponds across the road and planted them with salmon, which he later released in the canal. He was careful about the activities he chose, however: No wood-chopping, because as a surgeon he really needed all of his fingers.

A very sad thing happened at the Canal in 1919. One of the Nordstrom girls, Mabel, who was fourteen years old, went hiking in the woods with her family and drank water from a contaminated stream. As a result she became very ill with typhoid fever, and died of it. It was a great tragedy for the Nordstrom family and for their friends at the Canal, as we were like a large extended family up there.

Bud Hallberg, whose father developed the Hood Canal property, has been on the Board at Swedish for many years, as his father was before him. Bud has many happy memories of Hood Canal. He remembers that my father bought me a Welsh pony and a little two-wheeled cart. There was a small steamer that hauled freight to Union City on the Canal, so Father had the pony and cart shipped in for me to use during the summer.

Here's how Bud described the pony's arrival:

"Lloyd Nordstrom and I were just kids, maybe 10 years old. Doc Johanson had a big riding horse he kept up there. He asked Lloyd and me to drive the little pony and cart back to his place from Union City (about two miles), and he rode his horse. The pony had blinders on. Lloyd and I got in the cart, and we didn't know anything about horses. Away we go. Then Doctor Johanson would ride up behind us, cloppity-clop. The little pony would hear that and he would stop, because he couldn't see what was coming. Or an automobile would come up behind us. The pony would stop and start to back up, and we'd have a lot of trouble getting him moving again.

Finally we got the doctor to drop back. But when we went to turn in the gate at his property we didn't know how to handle the pony. He started to back up again, and backed right into a big drainage ditch. Lloyd fell out into the mud. That little pony was strong, and he clawed his way up out of the ditch and pulled the cart right up with him. Kitty enjoyed having the pony cart, and used to ride it around up there a lot. They had other horses too. One was a big black horse named Major. Lloyd and I used to bathe that horse in Hood Canal. We had an awful time getting him into the water, but once he got in he enjoyed it so much that we had an awful time getting him out."

Bud's account brought back many happy memories of the fun I had with my pony cart. During the summer we children would get as brown as berries and as tough as nails from all the exercise. Life in Seattle seemed very remote for that two or three month period. But inevitably Labor Day rolled around and it was time to head back to our home in the city. I can remember those sad feelings as summer drew to a close, but there was also some excitement about getting back home again.

After we spent three or four summers at the Canal as tent dwellers my father had a house built, with all the conveniences such as electricity and indoor plumbing. I'm sure my mother appreciated the less rigorous way of life, but I kind of missed the tenting days.

Later on when Elmer and I were married, Hood Canal continued to be a part of our life. I still spend several months there each summer.

My father and the other board members who had Hood Canal property thought it would be nice to have a picnic there for the class of graduating nurses on the hospital staff and this became an annual affair for many years. Mother and the other wives would set up big tables outdoors for a picnic lunch, and the young nurses enjoyed swimming and boating and beachcombing.

The event gradually evolved into a Swedish Hospital staff picnic.

Even after I was grown up and married, the picnic continued to be held and it became a family affair to which we all brought our children. Later on the picnic outgrew that location. A similar outing was held for the Nordstrom shoe store staff for many years, but it also grew too large for the Canal, so later they held their picnics at places like Beaver Lake, near Issaquah.

Hood Canal played a very important part in my father's life. Even though he was always busy up there with his various projects, still it was a break from the pressure of managing the hospital and his surgical practice. It gave him a chance to get away from the problems of his demanding medical career and enjoy family life in a way he could not do in the city. I cherish the memories of those good times with my parents and our friends. Hood Canal played an important role in my life for another reason, because that is where I first met my husband.

My parents continued to use their vacation home at Hood Canal until they sold their property during World War II. Mother didn't stay there much unless I was with her. Country life really wasn't her favorite thing. When our boys were youngsters I used to take them up there for about three weeks in the summer, but I didn't like to leave Elmer for the entire summer.

A man named Middleton from Aberdeen filled in the small bay next to my parents' property and put in a big bulkhead. He built a year-round house, with five bedrooms, five baths, and a furnace. Elmer and I bought the house from him about 25 years ago. It's 100 feet from the water. At about that time our son John bought a house just two doors from us. Illsley Nordstrom (Lloyd's widow) now owns the house my parents built.

Donol Hedlund, our old friend from boating days, has a house just down the road from us. So we have a nice little community of our own there.

After Elmer's retirement we began to spend the winter months in Palm Desert, California, and part of the time at our condominium at Madison Park, continuing to spend our summers at Hood Canal. Since Elmer's death in 1993 I have divided my year in much the same fashion. I particularly enjoy visits from our children and grandchildren during my stay on Hood Canal. When summer comes I still get that feeling of eager anticipation for life on the beach that I had so long ago when we piled our belongings in Father's car and embarked on the daylong journey to Hood Canal. These days the trip takes only about two hours!

Chapter Eight

Through Troubled Years

I f you look at the pattern of growth which Swedish Hospital established from its inception, you can see a reflection of my father's continual quest for excellence. He was determined that the hospital would be equipped to keep pace with important medical milestones as they occurred.

The practice of medicine was in a state of tremendous change at the time Swedish Hospital was founded, because of a series of important discoveries. Where previously kitchen table surgery had been performed in the patient's home, medical practice was now becoming office and hospital based. The role of the hospital had been revolutionized by 1900. Special facilities had to be provided for the housing of x-ray machines and laboratories. Sterile operating rooms were necessary for the greatly increased number of surgical cases.

In 1875 there were 661 hospitals in the United States, but by 1900 this number had tripled. Between 1900 and 1929, hospitals were opened at the rate of 200 per year. When Swedish opened its doors in 1910, it was one of 129 hospitals in the state of Washington. It soon emerged as a leader among these because of my father's determination to provide the highest quality of skills and equipment needed for the optimum practice of medicine.

Two years after moving to the Summit and Columbia location, provision was made for improved nurses' quarters. The Sanderson residence at Columbia and Minor was purchased at a cost of $30,000 and the Rininger home was moved across the alley to be annexed to this residence, providing living quarters for 50 nurses.

In 1916 an additional $85,000 was spent to build a 60-bed modern addition to the hospital, making a total of 100 beds. When money was required for such purposes it was raised through bank credit, mortgages, and small-denomination bonds.

The hospital laboratory of today is a domain of itself. Skilled technicians deal with intricate equipment which provides a tremendous variety of test results. During the first few years that Swedish Hospital was in operation, however, staff doctors did all their own lab work in a small laboratory provided in the hospital. This entailed long hours for the medical staff.

The Standardization Committee (forerunner of the present Executive Committee) was established to maintain the highest ethical standards. My father was one of the original members of this committee of doctors, who met once a month to discuss any deaths which had occurred in the hospital, and to talk about new treatments which evolved.

An important medical milestone at this point was the production of a tetanus antitoxin. Its introduction coincided with our country's entry into World War I in 1917, and it undoubtedly saved the lives of many wounded soldiers. If we step on a rusty nail we take it for granted that a tetanus booster shot will protect us from further problems. Prior to 1917, however, even a minor injury could bring on a tortured and terrible death from tetanus, or "lockjaw," as it often was called because of one of its more terrifying symptoms.

With the war years and the movement of troops throughout Europe, another extreme threat to health appeared on the horizon — the influenza epidemic of 1918, from which many thousands of persons died throughout the world. It was a particularly virulent form of flu, and those who came down with it were quite likely to die. There were no sulfa drugs and no antibiotics of any kind in 1918.

I was a little girl at the time of the flu epidemic, but I remember that we all wore gauze masks at any public gathering, and there was a great deal of fear of this illness. Many Seattle families had lost members or friends to the disease. The epidemic created greatly overcrowded conditions at Swedish Hospital. Fortunately, Doctor Carl Leede had gone through a previous flu epidemic in Hamburg. He instituted at Swedish the treatment which had met with a high degree of success in Germany, with good results.

Windows were kept closed. Patients were rubbed with camphorated oil and wrapped in sweat-packs, and each room had its container of boiling water and Eucalyptus oil. The hospital smelled like a Eucalyptus forest. At first the nurses voiced objections to the continuous nasal assault, but as the nurses themselves began to come down with the flu and learned at first hand how the vapors helped their breathing, fewer complaints were heard. This treatment saved many lives.

During the height of the epidemic, Swedish admitted only maternity patients and emergency surgical patients. Fathers and other family members were not allowed to visit the maternity floors, so nurses served as go-betweens. A father waiting in the lobby had to take the nurse's word that his brand new son was one of the cutest babies she had ever seen. Nurses who had trained at Swedish were commended for their treatment of a later flu epidemic in Alaska.

The decade following World War I was a prosperous one for the country, and Seattle underwent a period of unprecedented growth. Swedish Hospital took a major step in 1926 by building a seven-story fireproof addition, at a cost of $300,000. This brought the hospital's capacity up to 200 beds and 45 bassinets. I remember the grand opening celebration of this addition, and how happy my father and other Board members were to be able to offer this wonderful new facility to the public.

Everything about the hospital's progress seemed aligned on a straight path of accomplishment and improvement, but there was trouble waiting in the wings. I think it is fortunate that we can't see in advance when a dark cloud is about to descend, or we might not have the courage to face it.

The trouble in store was, of course, the Great Depression, which began with the stock market crash of 1929. The economy of the entire country was suddenly sent into a tailspin. Unemployment was rampant, and breadlines appeared in cities. This was not the kind of temporary economic setback our country has experienced from time to time over the years. It was instead a chill wind which blew throughout the land and extinguished the hopes and dreams of Americans. I remember driving by the row of flimsy shacks occupied by homeless unemployed men. That area of Seattle was known as Hooverville, because many blamed the Depression on the policies of President Herbert Hoover.

Our family was not affected in the drastic way that many others were during the depression but there was an undercurrent of distress because of my father's concern about the hospital and its employees. The patient load dropped precipitously, as sick people postponed needed hospitalization and surgery unless an emergency occurred. The beautiful new six-story addition was sparsely populated now, and several floors were closed to cut down on expenses. My father and fellow Board members worried about mortgage payments, and perhaps regretted their optimism in entering into the major expansion of 1926.

The Great Depression showed no signs of releasing its icy hold on the nation. Swedish Hospital entered into its most perilous period as Board members faced the difficult task of letting valued employees go in order to meet the hospital's payroll. The period of austerity was to extend past the mid-thirties. Cutting back and doing without became a way of life for the majority of the nation's population. Those were dark days indeed.

Chapter Nine

On My Own

Although Chapter Eight ended on a down note, we know from the present eminent position of Swedish Medical Center that it weathered its darkest moments successfully.

I need to go back now to the years following World War I. I've already told you that 1920 marked the beginning of many happy years in which my father and I shared our interest in horseback riding. But when I reached the teen years my interest shifted from horses to automobiles. In those days you could drive a car if you were fourteen years old. I could hardly wait for that birthday to roll around, because Father had promised me a car. I went with him to pick it out, and can still remember how wonderful it looked in the dealer's showroom. It was a two-toned beige Nash with a rumble seat. Although it was called a roadster then, it was the equivalent of a convertible.

I guess all of us remember our first car with much affection. As soon as I slipped behind the wheel of my

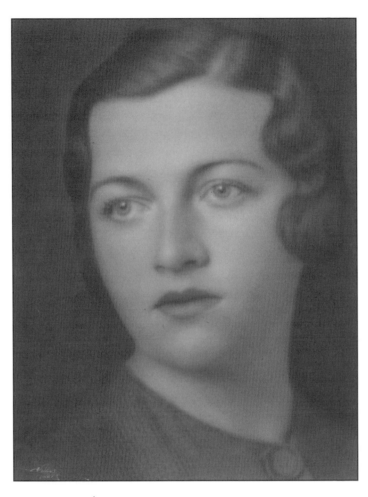

This rather soulful picture was taken just before my wedding.

sporty little roadster I knew that life from then on couldn't help but be pretty exciting. It wasn't only the car that changed my life. Father had finally let me forego the tutor and return to a school situation. I attended one year at Miss Ransom's in California, but then came home and finished high school at St. Nicholas, a private school for girls which was on Capitol Hill, where we lived. I enjoyed my years there very much because of the companionship of the other girls.

Although my parents could well afford to send me to college, I was not at all interested in any further schooling at that time. I was anxious to find out if I could support myself. I'm afraid this was a disappointment to my father, because he had a particular ambition for me. He wanted me to become a pediatrician! I was just beginning to discover who I was, however, and I wanted to plan my own life. This carried me along to the next step, which was to get a job.

Even though the Depression still prevailed, somehow I managed to find employment as a case worker for the Washington State Emergency Relief. My job was to call on families in need of assistance, to verify their situation. I was assigned to a territory in Ballard, and with a good Swedish name like Johanson I was welcomed warmly in that Scandinavian community.

I was only about 20 or 21, but I must have been good at my job as I was offered a similar job in Everett with a larger territory, and I moved there in 1932. I had continued to live at home while working in Seattle, but now I moved into a boarding house in Everett and thought that was a wonderful way to live. Because I was an only child I had been more or less hovered over as I grew up, and I was thrilled to be on my own at last.

My father had mixed feelings about the life he would like his daughter to pursue. He had told me of his hope that I might become a pediatrician, which certainly would have involved my leaving home. Yet when I told him of my plan to accept the Everett job and move to the boarding house he seemed very disappointed, and said he had hoped I would remain living at home as a companion to my mother. I had, however, apparently inherited his enthusiasm for the challenge of new frontiers. I think he recognized this finally, and bowed to my decision to leave home.

As it turned out, my years as a career girl were numbered because before long romance entered the picture. I have told you that during my childhood summers at Hood Canal my good friend had been Lloyd Nordstrom, as we were the same age. His older brother, Elmer, was seven years older than I was. When you are twelve years old and a young man is nineteen, he might as well be forty-one as far as common interests are concerned. When you become a young lady of fifteen, however, and the young man is an attractive 22 year old college senior, then he becomes of far greater interest. At least that's the way it was for me.

Apparently Elmer had noticed that I was no longer that little tomboy friend of his younger brother's. When I was fifteen years old I was very surprised to receive a call from Elmer Nordstrom asking if I would like to attend a formal dance given by Beta Theta Pi, his fraternity at the University of Washington. Because my parents knew Elmer and his family so well they were quite willing for me to attend the dance with him, and there was a great flurry about finding just the right formal dress to wear.

On the night of the party when Elmer arrived, looking handsome in his tuxedo and bearing a corsage for me, I felt completely grown up and in an exciting new social milieu. My confidence was short-lived however. When we got to the dance I was by far the youngest girl there, and the other girls chose to totally ignore me. For that reason the evening was not a great success for me, but still it was nice to get to know Elmer as someone other than just Lloyd's big brother. I'm not going to tell you that the Beta formal was the beginning of our romance, as we didn't really begin dating until much later—when I was out of school and earning my living as a case worker.

When Elmer came around again at that time showing obvious interest in me, there was no question but that we now were on an equal footing as grownups, and on that basis our friendship gradually turned into love. When he proposed marriage I accepted, but there was one more hurdle that was expected of him. He needed to ask my parents' permission to marry me.

Although their approval was readily given, Elmer had the feeling my father actually had expected a great deal more for me in the way of a prospective husband. "After all," Elmer told me, "I was just a shoe clerk then and you were his pride and joy." I think he probably was wrong about that, as my parents knew his family so well and had known Elmer since he was just a boy. I'm sure

Father thought I had made a good choice. After all, Elmer was Swedish. That must have counted for quite a few points in his favor!

We were married in 1934, when I was 23 and Elmer was 30. We had a lovely wedding at my parents' home. I believe there were about fifty guests, with a reception in the third floor party room. I wore a beautiful long white bridal gown which was trimmed with rosepoint lace from my mother's wedding dress. I'm sorry to say I can't remember what Elmer wore!

We went on our honeymoon to the World's Fair in Chicago. They were assembling Chevrolets at the Fair, and we bought one. We stayed in Chicago two or three days while they got our car ready. Then we drove to Milwaukee, where we visited relatives of my family. While we were there Elmer did some business with the Nunn Bush shoe company. Then we drove to Montreal and Quebec, and back down through New England to New York, where we had some dear friends. In Elmer's autobiography he said we visited every shoe store in New York City. He called it a typical Nordstrom honeymoon, because it seemed that with the three Nordstrom brothers the shoe business was never very far from their minds. Then we headed west, stopping in Denver to see my mother's family, and then home. We were gone about a month, and shoe stores or not, I thought it was a lovely honeymoon.

After our marriage Elmer and my father became very good friends. They were real buddies and used to have long discussions, sometimes strongly disagreeing. But it was obvious that they enjoyed and respected each other.

In 1937 he was invited to join the Board of Swedish Hospital. He was the youngest member but he had the respect of the other Board members. They had known him since he was a young boy, as many of them had summer homes at Hood Canal.

When Elmer and I were married I quit my job, as that seemed to be what young women did in those days. My career became that of a homemaker, and before too long, a mother. We bought a house on Capitol Hill for $7,000, an amount that was a little scary for us but it was an awfully good buy. It was at 911 Eleventh Avenue East, two blocks south of Volunteer Park. We lived there for ten years. In 1937 our first son, John Nils Nordstrom, was born. He was named John for Elmer's father, and Nils for mine. James Frederick Nordstrom came along in 1940. Both boys were of course born at Swedish Hospital.

My parents were delighted to have grandchildren. I can remember how excited Father was when John's birth was imminent. Board member or not, he wasn't permitted in the delivery room. I was told that he lingered outside the door and was just about beside himself until word was received that I was fine and had given birth to a healthy little boy. Incidentally, my having a baby of my own did not change my father's lifelong habit of calling me Baby. I don't ever remember his calling me Katharine or Kitty. It was always just Baby. When I was a little girl and we went riding together, the English grooms called me Miss Baby. (Father called my mother Kate, and she always called him Doctor. Most of his friends called him Jo, and his relatives in Sweden called him August.)

That time around 1940 was a very happy period for our family. Elmer and I were enjoying our two young sons, and my parents doted on them. The country had finally emerged from the Depression years, and we did not know that World War II was just ahead of us. My father's life was active as ever, combining his responsibilities as a busy surgeon and his role in spearheading the continued progress which maintained Swedish Hospital in a position of leadership.

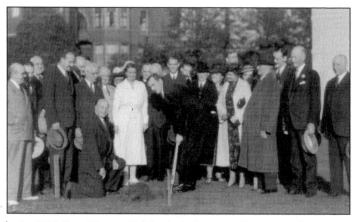

In 1938 Gov. Clarence D. Martin broke ground for a new wing at Swedish Hospital. My father is on his knees. Next to him is Herina Eklind, RN, who was Director of Nursing and then superintendent of the hospital for many years.

Chapter Ten

Leaving Dark Days Behind

In 1928 my father had attended an international congress on cancer in London, and he was struck with the tremendous need for research and treatment for this disease. Even though the discovery of radium had taken place only a few years before, the effect of irradiation on cancer cells had already been noted and was the subject of considerable study in Sweden. My father was in touch with these developments, and was determined to involve Swedish Hospital in the battle against cancer.

By 1932 the Depression was firmly entrenched and its limiting effect upon the hospital continued. How typical of my father's optimism and foresight that despite the era of austerity, he chose that year to establish the Swedish Hospital Tumor Institute. At his urging, the Board commissioned Carl F. Gould, the city's most prominent architect, to draw plans for a new building to house the facility.

The Swedish Hospital Tumor Institute opened its doors in 1934, the only non-profit institute in the

Pacific Northwest devoted solely to the diagnosis and management of cancer. Its prestige has continued to grow and it has achieved worldwide renown and respect for its high standards of research and care.

Meanwhile improvements continued to be made to the hospital itself. In 1936 a new boiler house was constructed, as well as two new surgeries, a new laboratory and pharmacy, at a total cost of $92,000. The following year the orthopedic wing, including a swimming pool for water therapy, was built at a cost of $86,000, which increased the hospital's capacity to 250 beds. This wing was undertaken especially for the treatment of crippled children under the auspices of the Welfare Department of the State of Washington.

By now Father was in his sixties. One might expect that with increasing age he would become less venturesome in adding new facilities to the hospital. Not so. In 1941 a new modern nursery was completed, at a cost of $123,000, making a total of 75 bassinets.

Most babies born at Swedish Hospital during the 1930's remained there for an average of five days, but one youngster stayed for three years! He was David Ishii, a Japanese baby whose mother died at his birth in 1935. He was the youngest of five children, and his father felt unable to take the infant into the motherless home. A little bending of the rules apparently went on, and the baby remained in the Swedish Hospital nursery. David's father took his older children to Japan to be cared for there. It was expected that in a few months the father would return to Seattle and be able to take the baby, but the months stretched into years. Meanwhile David remained in the nursery—a great favorite of the nurses.

When David was old enough to talk he was responsible for endowing my father with a nickname by which he would affectionately be referred to by most of the hospital staff members from that time on. Dr. Nils August Johanson was called "Papa Jo" by David Ishii, and Papa Jo he became to one and all, but seldom to his face.

One of the nurses, Ruth Ulleland, was largely responsible for David's care. When he was three years old she obtained his father's permission to board the little boy with her aunt and uncle, whose name was also Johanson (no relation to my family). They operated the Johanson berry farm at Cove, on Vashon Island, where he stayed for three years. At that time David's father returned to Seattle and remarried. A young stepmother took over the raising of David and his brothers and sisters. As a young man David sometimes returned to the hospital to visit the nurses he had become fond of during his stay there. For some years now he has been the proprietor of a popular bookstore in the Pioneer Square area. He reports that he has a list of about twenty nurses who have dropped into his bookstore to tell him they remember when he was the star boarder of the Swedish Hospital nursery.

The nursery has entertained its share of celebrities throughout the years. In 1939 the hospital was honored with visits from Mrs. Eleanor Roosevelt, then First Lady of the land, when her daughter Anna gave birth to a son. Anna's husband at that time was John Boettiger, who was publisher of the Seattle Post-Intelligencer. During her visit Mrs. Roosevelt became a staunch supporter of the Swedish Hospital Tumor Institute, and used her influence on its behalf from time to time.

A large hospital continually serves as the background for real-life drama, and Swedish Hospital is no exception. There have been the usual number of maternity cases arriving at the hospital so late that the baby is born in the hospital courtyard. One unusual incident involved a 30-year old gypsy princess who was undergoing a serious operation at the hospital. One hundred of the young woman's tribesmen came from California and Oregon to be with their princess, and all of them gathered in the hospital's lobby during her operation. The gypsy women, wearing long colorful gowns and heavy costume jewelry, created a vivid picture as they waited to learn that the operation had been successful.

In 1931 the original Rininger wing of the hospital was razed, and a new building constructed at a cost of $352,000. The four pillars from the original Rininger residence, which had been incorporated in the old entrance, were moved to the garden of the nurses' home which was completed in 1946 at a cost of $450,000.

Eklind Hall (which later became a part of the Fred Hutchinson Research Institute) provided living quarters for 120 nurses, and contained classrooms, offices, laboratories, and an auditorium. The main lounge featured a beautiful Swedish modern fireplace. Each floor had its own lounge with Pullman kitchen.

This was a project in which my father had a particular interest. He had recognized the importance of excellent nursing care from the very early days of that first small hospital on Belmont Avenue, and he established the school of nursing as an important adjunct to the hospital. He had a sincere interest in the educational program for the nursing students, but also a warm regard for the welfare of these young women. The new nurses' home grew out of his desire to provide them with attractive and comfortable living quarters during their training period.

Eklind Hall was built on property purchased from James Daniel Lowman, a pioneer stationer in Seattle. He and his wife had planted a young walnut tree at their former home in the East in 1881. They later transplanted the tree to the garden of their Seattle residence. When the property was sold to Swedish Hospital (to be available upon his death) Mr. Lowman asked that the tree not be cut. A brick wall was built around the court of Eklind Hall, and bricklayers formed the wall around a low branch of the tree, leaving a circular opening around the branch.

I've always thought there is something very satisfying about planting a tree, the general expectation being that the tree will continue living long after we're gone. For that reason I'm sorry to report that the walnut tree eventually gave way to the expansion of the hospital facilities. But in a way it still survives. Doctor Alan Lobb, who served as Medical Director and then Executive Director of Swedish Medical Center for 27 years, is a talented artist. On the day the walnut tree came down, Dr. Lobb was on hand to rescue most of the wood, some of which he carved into beautiful works of art. Among the items he made from the walnut wood were beautiful gavels for each Board member. Knowing the history of that tree, my husband was particularly pleased with this gift.

Chapter Eleven

All in the Family

Throughout the years there have been many additions and revisions to buildings which house Swedish Medical Center. This might have resulted in a hodge-podge effect had it not been for Swedish's long association with the distinguished architectural firm of Naramore, Bain, Brady & Johanson. Their skilled services have provided a unifying influence, with particular attention to careful blending of the new with the old. It sometimes has been a difficult decision as to whether a particular structure should be updated or removed to make way for a more efficient building. The Board's focus on such problems has been greatly facilitated by the advice received from knowledgeable architects.

My dear cousin, the late Perry Johanson, was a founding partner of Naramore, Bain, Brady and Johanson. His outstanding architectural skills were already evident while he was still in college, at which time he won an award from the A.I.A. to study in Paris.

These portraits of my father's parents were done by his brother Erik, who was a Northwest artist.

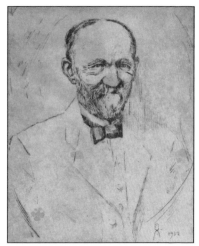

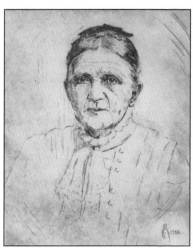

My father was very fond of Perry. He was so pleased about the award that he augmented it with a financial gift of his own which enabled Perry to double his stay in Paris.

When Perry returned to the University of Washington after his stay in France, his studies included a class in sculpture and there he met an attractive young artist named Jean Peterson (also Swedish). Their mutual interests and background led to friendship and then to a very happy marriage. Their family included a daughter, Kristina, and a son, Peter.

Shortly after Perry began his architectural practice in Seattle, Swedish Hospital was about to undertake one of its expansions. My father persuaded the Board that Perry would be a good choice as the architect. Any concern about nepotism was quickly dispelled once the work was completed. Perry did such an outstanding job that he soon was greatly in demand to provide architectural services for other hospitals. Among these were Providence Hospital, the Veterans Administration Hospital, and the University of Washington Health Sciences Center and Teaching Hospital. He completed additional projects for Swedish, and when he became a partner in NBBJ in 1946, that firm began its long and mutually advantageous relationship with the medical center.

Nels Johanson, Perry's older brother, became the president of Pioneer Sand and Gravel, and served on the board at Swedish for a time.

Jean Johanson continued her work as a sculptor and designer of mosaics. She has completed important commissions, such as for Portland's Lloyd Center, and her work can be found in many private collections. Perry and Jean had a home in the Hilltop area of Bellevue for many years. While they were on a visit to Spokane in 1981, Perry suffered a heart attack and died. Jean later moved to Covenant Shores, the retirement community on Mercer Island. Perry and I were good friends and I remember him very fondly.

My father's brother Erik must have been particularly proud of his son's achievement as an architect because he was himself a gifted artist. Although trained as a tailor, at which he worked for many years, his true love was in the field of fine arts. He was a founding member of the Pacific Northwest Painters Group, made up of the area's most talented artists, and his work was of prize-winning quality. He was a good friend of Eustace Ziegler, the famous painter of Alaskan scenes, and they often went on painting expeditions together. Elmer and I particularly enjoy one of Erik's paintings which we have on display at Hood Canal. It won an award at a showing at the Seattle Art Museum.

One of my cousins, Swen Swenson (son of Father's sister Rika), has portraits which Erik painted of my grandparents. Swen lives in Lake Oswego, Oregon. He is close to my age. He lived in Lund, Sweden until the age of six, when he and his parents came to this country. They went first to Index, Washington, where Erik Johanson had a general store. Swen's father, Elof Swenson, worked in Erik's store for a year or so. My father visited his relatives in Index, and Swen remembers that as a small boy he was particularly impressed that my father drove up in a big Packard Twin Six. At the time the Swenson family lived in Index, Father's sister Anna and her husband, Max Schertle, also lived there. Max was principal of the local school.

Swen married Ruth Backstrom, a Swedish girl who was born in this country, and they have two children, both of whom have interesting careers. Their daughter, Karen, is a fine musician who has played first violin with the Seattle Symphony for about thirty years. Her husband, Robert Bonnevie, plays first French horn with the Symphony. Swen's son, Neil, who lives in Snoqualmie, Washington, is a Seattle police officer.

I'm proud of the accomplishments of all of my relatives, both here and in Sweden. I think my father's family is typical of all those Swedish immigrants who arrived in the Pacific Northwest at the turn of the century. They worked very hard to establish a new life here, sometimes against great odds. They saw to it that their children received the education which they had been denied, and those children now are making a valued contribution to this community.

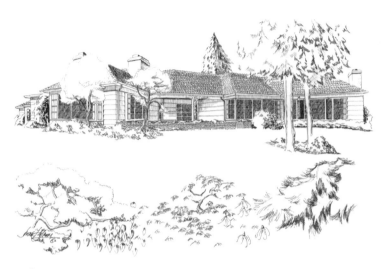

Elmer and I raised our two sons
in this Windermere house, which
we loved.

Chapter Twelve

Letting Go the Reins

In about 1940 my parents sold the house on Capitol Hill, and moved to a house on the north end of Lake Washinton. They only lived there for a few years, however. In 1944 my mother, who had always been such a healthy person, developed a heart problem and after being seriously ill for less than a month she died. Father was just lost without her. His busy career as a surgeon and hospital administrator had prevented him from spending as much time with her as he would have liked. I am sure they both felt that in the retirement years there would be more time to do the things together they had looked forward to, but this was not to be.

At the time of my mother's death the new nurses' home, Eklind Hall, was nearing completion. The many details of this project helped to take my father's mind off his loss, but still he was very lonely. After my mother's death he sold the house they had moved to, but couldn't seem to decide upon another living arrangement. He

Our sons, James and John, were very fond of their grand- father, and he loved them very much.

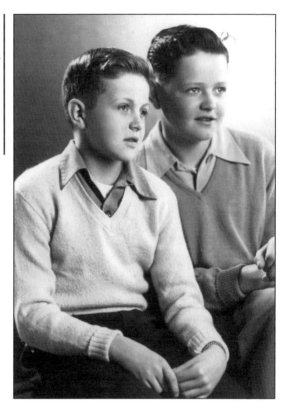

considered buying a house in Windermere, but eventually decided against it. Elmer and I had admired the house when Father was looking at it, and after he ruled it out for himself we decided to buy it. That was in 1944. Our family loved that house and we owned it for more than forty years, until Elmer and I bought our condominium at Madison Park. It was a wonderful place for the boys to grow up. They had lots of neighborhood friends, and there was swimming and boating nearby. The Lloyd Nordstroms lived across the street, on the water, so the boys had a boat there, and did a lot of waterskiing.

Father continued to search for a comfortable home for himself, but of course the essential ingredient for that was missing now that my mother was gone. The parents of Illsley Ball Nordstrom (Lloyd's wife) had moved into a suite in the Olympic Hotel, and my father tried that for a while, but he was not happy there. His own health was failing at that time, and eventually he moved into the hospital. In 1944 he gave up his private practice of surgery, but remained as President of the Board at the hospital. Retirement was not easy for him. He had always been such a steamer, and it was very difficult for him to let go of the reins and leave things to others in charge.

By 1946 Father's heart condition was quite serious, and he had a nurse who looked after him. She used to drive him out to our house several times a week to have dinner and enjoy the boys. Jim and John were six and nine years old then, and he was crazy about them. They loved him very much too. When they heard his car arrive out in back they would make a run for it to see who could get to Grandpa first and help him into the house. He loved those little boys so much that I'm really sorry he didn't live long enough to see what fine men they became. He would have been so proud of all they have accomplished.

In June of 1946 my father resigned as President of the Board of Swedish Hospital. In October he suffered a fatal heart attack and died in the hospital he had founded. He was seventy-four years old. When news spread throughout the hospital that he had passed away, there were saddened hearts among the many staff members who had known and loved "Papa Jo."

My mother's death had been very hard on him, and he lived only two years after that. His passing was very sad for me even though I had known that with his serious heart condition he might not be with us much longer. The death of a parent is never easy to accept, expected as it may be.

The nineteen men who served as pallbearers and honorary pallbearers at his funeral included his good friends who had put up the original money for the founding of Swedish Hospital, fellow Board members, and many of the doctors who had been original staff members.

The newspaper obituary described him as the guiding spirit of Swedish Hospital. It stated that at the time of his death he was a member of the American College of Surgeons, King County Medical Association, Rainier Club, Men's University Club, Washington Athletic Club, and Swedish Business Men's Club. He had previously been president of the Seattle Hospital Council.

The day after his death a letter addressed to my father arrived from the King of Sweden advising that he was to be awarded the order of the Northern Star for his work in founding Swedish Hospital and his leadership in bringing the hospital to prominence in the medical community. My father was very proud of being a Swede, and loved the land of his birth. He would have been so pleased to be chosen for this honor. Unfortunately, the Northern Star is not awarded posthumously, so with his death the opportunity to receive it had passed. I feel honored, however, that he had been selected for this decoration. When I think of my father's perseverance in coming to this country as a very young man, working hard to achieve his ambition to become a physician, and then undertaking the mammoth task of building a hospital complex, I think he was more than deserving of the honor from the King of Sweden.

Sometimes a successful organization will fall apart upon the death of its founder. It is a measure of my father's foresight that he set up procedures which would endure beyond his life span, so that the hospital would continue its pattern of excellence and growth after he was gone.

Several months after Father's passing, my husband was named president of the Board of Directors of Swedish Hospital. Elmer felt especially confident in accepting this responsibility because during the preceding year he and my father had held many conversations on the subject of the hospital's future. In a way Father seemed to be handing over the reins to someone he loved and trusted. Elmer knew exactly the direction in which Father hoped the hospital would proceed. In the years that followed he and his fellow Board members were able to make many of those goals a reality. In later years Elmer became a life member of the Board, which meant he was welcome to take part in Board meetings but was not required to be there. Whenever we were in Seattle, however, he enjoyed participating in decisions and his contact with the Board continued until his death. Our son Jim continues the family tradition as a Board member. I have an idea there will be Nordstroms showing up on that Board for many years to come!

*My parents,
after my father
had retired.*

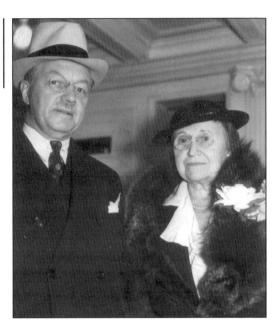

Chapter Thirteen

A Labor of Love

S wedish Medical Center is such a going concern these days that it's hard to imagine that its future could ever have been in doubt. But the history of hospitals founded in Seattle and elsewhere is replete with examples of those which went out of existence after a comparatively short life. I think the secret of success during the early days of Swedish lay in the fact that my father was not only a strong leader, but a very farsighted man. He always had a picture in mind of what the hospital could be in years to come, and was never content to sit back and let things coast for a while.

Since his passing, the Board of Trustees deserves much credit for its ability to find administrators who have had that same eye toward the future. When Dr. Alan Lobb became Medical Director and then Executive Director, arriving in 1961, he began immediately to demonstrate that it was not enough to continue in the successful mode of the present. Time after time he brought before the Board new projects which at first may have seemed a little too far out for a rather conservative institution to inaugurate.

The Elmer Nordstrom Tower is a good example. Office condominiums for physicians? Who had ever heard of that? At first the idea met with resistance from those it was designed to benefit most—the physicians. But Dr. Lobb persisted, the Board went along with him, and the medical community has benefited greatly from his vision. If there had been such a building in my father's day, I'm sure he would have been the first to purchase one of the units, knowing the amount of time he could save in his busy day if he were able to walk across a sky bridge from his clinical office to the hospital.

Back in 1962 I received a telephone call from Dr. Lobb, with a special invitation. He asked me to lunch to discuss forming a women's auxiliary. I told him I'd be happy to help get it organized, which I did. I would like to give full credit to a group of doctors' wives, who sent letters to prominent women in the community asking them to join. One of those founders of the Swedish Medical Center Auxiliary is Mrs. Joan Sanderson, whose late husband, Dr. Eric Sanderson, was a former Chief of Staff at Swedish. Mrs. Sanderson has been a tireless worker on behalf of the hospital. She has been in charge of the very profitable gift shop which the Auxiliary operates in the hospital lobby since its inception, first as a volunteer and later as a professional. In recent years she has become the first woman member of the hospital's Board of Trustees.

While I have not been active in the day-to-day operation of the Auxiliary, I have enjoyed contributing what I could in the way of moral support. Every fall for more than 30 years I hosted a luncheon for the Auxiliary's volunteers. They were encouraged to bring as guests any friends who might be interested in joining the Auxiliary. It was always a lovely occasion, and we had a special "oldtimers' table" for old friends who had retired from the nursing staff.

The Auxiliary is now under the direction of a professional director. An awards luncheon is held each spring in recognition of its volunteers. Several volunteers have contributed in excess of 15,000 hours. I think that's remarkable!

The nice thing is that our volunteers enjoy their work so much. Someone may move to Seattle and not know many people. A friend might say, "Well, I volunteer at Swedish Hospital. Why don't you come along and see how you like it?" I've had so many women say to me after they've been working as volunteers for two or three years, "You know, I have made the most wonderful friends. I don't know what I would have done in Seattle if I hadn't started as a volunteer."

One of the Auxiliary activities which I find particularly appealing and valuable is the cuddler program, in which volunteers visit the neonatal department to rock the babies. Premature infants must remain in the hospital for a matter of months. Often their families live in another city, so the tender loving care provided the infants by volunteers is truly appreciated.

Another important program is the work which volunteers do on behalf of the hospital's AIDS patients, helping out in any way they are needed in the unit, visiting with patients, providing magazines, etc. You also see the volunteers in their cheerful pink smocks as they assist discharged patients in leaving the hospital.

I'm particularly pleased that we have our Candy-stripers, the teen-age volunteers who come in during the summer. They are so enthusiastic and willing. Some of them work as many as three days a week, and come back for several years. The Auxiliary director writes a lot of college and job references for these youngsters, who have demonstrated their desire to be of service to others. The Candy-stripers have so much fun working at the hospital that they are very successful in recruiting their friends as volunteers.

The Auxiliary members also are responsible for a sizeable amount of money donated to the hospital each year. Their gift shop, which is tastefully and expertly stocked by Joan Sanderson, raises a considerable amount of money for the hospital. Perhaps most important of all, each year the volunteers donate many thousands of hours of service. I'm so proud of them, and very appreciative of their efforts.

Chapter Fourteen

They Remember Him Fondly

One retired employee has been particularly active in planning reunion activities and keeping in touch with the friends he made during his employment at Swedish. Paul Baker (now 82), began working at Swedish in 1937 as an orderly when he was 24 years old. For many years he was an indispensable member of the surgical team. A great gentle bear of a man, at 6'4-1/2", he radiated his concern for surgical patients in a manner which endeared him to all. Instead of the usual way of transferring the patient from gurney to operating table, Paul would simply put his arms around the patient in a big hug and lift the patient carefully onto the table. "It seemed to kind of comfort them," he said.

One prominent Seattle woman underwent several surgeries at Swedish. When she was assigned another orderly to transport her to the operating room she flatly refused to go until she could be taken there by Paul Baker. In appreciation, her family later made a very generous gift to the medical center. I'm sure Paul's kindness contributed to the favorable impression which this family gained of Swedish. Paul has many memories of my father, having worked closely with him in surgery.

"If Dr. Johanson had to reprimand someone," said Paul, "he would do it quietly. And if you did good work, he showed his appreciation. Miss Tysdale was superintendent of the nursing staff in the operating room. She was really rough on the student nurses. If she knew they were going out on a date she would give them a lot of extra work to do—you know, scrubbing this and scrubbing that. All the girls were scared of her, and no wonder. If she didn't like something they did during surgery she would kick them under the table, and on some occasions she would even shake them. Well, I hadn't been there very long before she shook me one day. That did it! I went to Dr. Johanson and told him I was perfectly willing to take a bawling out, but no lady was going to shake me.

"His surprising reply was, 'Paul, I'm going to give you a $10 raise. I like what you do.' That made me feel better about the whole thing. I don't know what he said to Miss Tysdale, but I was never shaken again. Eventually Miss Tysdale married the brother of one of the nurses, and she seemed to mellow a whole lot after that."

Paul has a problem with his legs now, but gets around with a cane. For many years he went by bus to the downtown YMCA daily to swim, in order to keep his legs in as good shape as possible. He visits former

Swedish employees who are in nursing homes, and is active in keeping his old friends informed of what other retirees are doing. I think he is a wonderful example of the family spirit which my father always hoped to inspire in Swedish employees.

Each year Paul helps to make plans for the annual picnic at Woodland Park for retired Swedish employees and in 1995 there were 228 in attendance. Until just a few years ago, the picnic was always attended by Gertie Hytmo, who graduated from the Swedish school of nursing in 1918. When Gertie was well into her 90's, she continued to come down every year from Stanwood to attend the picnic, and also to attend the annual luncheon I gave for volunteers. It was always wonderful to see her.

Gertie remembered my father well. She too was impressed by the fact that he never lost his temper or said anything derogatory. "He never created a scene," she told me, "and believe me we had some doctors who did." Gertie laughed about my father's having so many things on his mind that he would get a trifle absent-minded. "We would hand him a list of his patients, then he would walk into the wrong room." She remembered him as a wonderful surgeon, who seemed also to have the knack of getting the very best doctors for his staff. "There was a saying among staff doctors," she said, "that anyone who couldn't get on the staff would give their eye teeth to get on it. There were a lot of applicants in those days, and I'm sure there still are."

Gertie kept in close touch with her old friend, Paul Baker, and called him every few days, until her death several years ago. The nurses with whom he worked were very fond of Paul. There is a reunion luncheon of retired nurses every two years, to which Paul is always invited. One year the group surprised him by making him the honored guest. Paul also helps with the annual Christmas luncheon for retirees. In December 1995 it was held at the Yankee Diner, with 75 in attendance.

Another retired employee who works closely with Paul Baker on retiree activities is Gunvor Thilberg, known as "Lindy" because her maiden name was Lindberg. She came to this country from Sweden at the age of ten, and after graduating from high school she came to Swedish in 1937 to work in the office. Eventually Lindy was made director of admitting and remained in that position for many years, retiring in 1978. Perhaps the best known anecdote about Lindy Thilberg concerns a jar in a paper sack which was left at the admitting desk for my father. Lindy was used to receiving specimens in this manner, and routinely sent it along to the lab. The analysis came back that the jar contained chicken soup. The woman who left it was the wife of a chef, who had prepared the soup as a treat for Father's lunch!

Lindy Thilberg remembers that my mother used to wait in the lobby for her husband to complete his rounds, and would chat with the admitting staff. "One time she confided in me that she wished the doctor would stay out of her garden," said Lindy, "as he really didn't know as much as he thought he did about gardening."

Lillian Clein, who died a few years ago, went to work in 1933 in the pharmacy department at Swedish. In fact,

Lillian was the pharmacy department, being its only employee. In an interview several years ago she remembered what a fine group of men the board members were. "They were all good business men in their field," said Lillian, "but they all deferred to Dr. Johanson. They knew he was the real spirit of the hospital. He was far ahead of his time. Whenever there was anything new, he was in the forefront and was willing to change things around in the hospital to accommodate the new idea if he thought it had merit. For example, I think we were the first ones around to have special rooms for allergy patients, where the atmosphere was controlled, and you couldn't have flowers, etc. No one else had even thought of that yet."

Lillian thought my father showed unusual skill not only in choosing doctors for the medical staff, but in selecting those who interned at the hospital. She remembered one young intern who was so bright and gifted that he stood out from all the others. "I told myself that here was a young doctor who was going to be someone special," she said. Lillian Clein was certainly correct in her assessment of the young intern. He was Doctor Ernest Burgess, the distinguished orthopedic surgeon whom you have already met in Chapter Six.

Lillian had offers to work elsewhere for more money, but loved working at Swedish. "It was such a democratic place to work," she said. "I remember the wonderful Christmas parties we had, where everyone from the maintenance staff to the superintendent just mingled and thoroughly enjoyed themselves. Dr. Johanson was always there, of course, and the other board members.

He was so well groomed and professional looking. I love the picture of him in the lobby. It looks exactly like him."

A retired nurse who remembers particularly the Depression years at Swedish is Dorothy Ditlefsen. She too joins in activities with her fellow retirees. I've known Dorothy for many years, and she was always an honored guest at my luncheon for volunteers. She was born at Swedish Hospital in 1912, and graduated from its school of nursing in 1934. Dorothy spent all but one year of her nursing career at Swedish, having worked for one year as a nurse in an industrial plant during World War II. She retired as head nurse of the Tumor Institute in 1980.

"During the Depression," Dorothy told me, "they had to let so many people go at the hospital that we student nurses were given a great deal of responsibility. You might have a whole floor by yourself at night." She told me that one night when she was on duty my father took her on a tour of the hospital to show her all of the fire doors and how they worked, and talked to her about what her response should be in the event of fire. "He also told me that if anyone ever wanted the cash box, to give it to them, and if someone was after narcotics, to give them what they wanted. 'Just don't get hurt,' was his advice to me. I really appreciated his taking the time to explain these things, which no one else had thought to tell me."

After she became an RN in 1934 Dorothy used to accompany my father on his rounds in the hospital. "I admired his skill," she said. "He really was a topnotch doctor, and his patients loved him. He was also a very interesting man to talk to, and during rounds he would talk to me about many different subjects. I remember that he told me it was important to hire good people and then leave them alone. He also said, 'Use the knowledge of your friends. If you know a banker, let him help you with your banking problems.' "

I guess that was another way in which my father was ahead of his times. These days they call that networking. Dorothy reminded me that my father always wore beautiful silk shirts, with his monogram on the sleeve. She remembers how nice he looked when he would come in to make rounds wearing his riding habit. I'm so glad we have the picture of Dad on horseback which I have included in this book.

Chapter Fifteen

A Travel Log

My father enjoyed travel, and did a lot of it in connection with management of Swedish Hospital. He visited many hospitals in this country to get ideas for improvements he wanted to make at Swedish. At one time he went to Vienna to study with a world-famous surgeon there. He also would go to Sweden to visit his family, but also to investigate innovations in the practice of medicine which were being tried in Sweden. He visited the Radiumhemmet in Sweden, where they were doing very advanced work with radiation therapy, and also attended a meeting in London in 1928 regarding cancer treatment. As a result he was inspired to establish the Swedish Hospital Tumor Institute in 1932.

On another occasion he visited Chicago when he heard that a hospital there had a one million volt x-ray tube, the only one in existence. He promptly ordered one for the Tumor Institute, and it was used for many years. I think part of it is in the Museum of History and Industry now. The disadvantage of x-ray for cancer therapy had been that people received terrible burns. The advantage of the million volt tube was that you could force the important rays through a filter so harmful rays did not get through and burn.

Much of the travel Elmer and I did was in connection with the Seahawks football team, when we were involved in its ownership. I don't recall my father having much interest in sports, although that may have been due to his heavy work schedule. I never showed much love for sports when I was growing up. That's why it still is surprising to me that for many years I attended close to twenty football games a year, and often had to fly across country to do it.

The Nordstroms became majority stockholders of the Seahawks in 1974, on the urging of Elmer's brother, Lloyd. Sadly, we lost Lloyd in January, 1974, shortly after he had accomplished his goal of bringing the NFL franchise to Seattle. The first owners' meeting after we acquired majority ownership was in March, 1974, at Coronado. After Lloyd's death it became Elmer's role to act as managing owner. All they had was a manager and a coach—no facilities and no players. Elmer had to help put the whole thing together, aided by the expertise of the other partners— Herman Sarkowsky, Lynn Himmelman, Monte Bean, Howard Wright and David Skinner.

From someone who had seldom watched a football game if I could help it, I became a fairly avid fan. It was fun traveling with the team, but it was hard work too. For the out of town games we would usually arrive the night before the game and go to the hotel. Some of us would probably have dinner together. The next morning, if we were in New York we'd get up at what would be 5 a.m. in Seattle, and go out to the stadium. After the game we'd sit in the bus and wait for the players to change their clothes. Then we'd head for the airport and start home—seven hours of flying time across the continent. And some planes had to stop for fuel, making the trip even longer.

We used Alaska Airlines for the last five or six years we had the team. They had a new plane coming out, so they painted the Seahawk logo on the nose. Their colors are the same as those of the Seahawks, blue and green. On the tail of the plane they had written in blue letters, "Seahawk One."

When someone would say to me, "Isn't it wonderful that you get to travel around the United States and see all these lovely places?" I'd say, "You know what I see? Airfields, insides of buses and stadiums. That's what I see!"

I don't mean to sound like I was not interested in the games. I was always happy when we won. I enjoyed a lot of the players. There were so many really wonderful young men involved, like Jim Zorn, Steve Largent, Dan Doornink. Dan put himself through medical school while he played football and is now practicing medicine. It was great knowing those young men, watching them play, and seeing them do well.

When the boys won they were full of songs and jokes and laughter on the trip home, and were a lot of fun to be around. If they didn't do well, that was another story. When they lost a game the gloom was so thick that you could cut it with a knife. After one particularly painful defeat I told Elmer the return flight was like a seven-hour funeral. I wonder whatever happened to "It matters not if you win or lose, it's how you play the game."

The Seahawks were a great responsibility for Elmer—as much responsibility, in fact, as running a very large business. And after all, he was supposed to be retired! For the final six or eight years that the family had the Seahawks, our son John took over as managing owner for the team.

Before the Seahawks interlude in our lives, Elmer and I did quite a bit of travelling around the world. We went to Europe four times, and on each trip we visited Sweden. It was wonderful to meet our relatives there, and to see the area in which my father had grown up. Lund is a lovely little town. I'm still in touch with my cousins in Sweden, and my cousin Signe (who has since passed away) provided me with some of the family names and dates for this book.

We thoroughly enjoyed England also, and visited Italy, France, Austria. We even went behind the iron curtain to Bratislava, in 1965. Czechoslovakia seemed a very sad place to me at that time, and it is so wonderful now to see how things have changed since we were there. I'm glad we made all those trips then. Traveling is hard work, and as you get older you don't want to have to cope with all the problems that can be involved.

Until I lost Elmer, we enjoyed traveling to the opening of each new Nordstrom store. They were so much fun! The openings are exciting, colorful and glamorous. There is usually a lovely buffet party the night before the store opens, sponsored by a charity which sells tickets to the party as a fund raiser. Nordstrom always provides a wonderful fashion show. Although we loved the openings, all members of the Nordstrom family who attended had to stand for three or four hours and visit with people at the reception. By the end of the evening my husband and I were really ready for a rest!

Wouldn't my father have been amazed at the success of the Nordstrom enterprises? We all are!

Chapter Sixteen

A Reputation Enhanced

E klind Hall was the final project my father accomplished at Swedish Hospital. The pattern he established of continued expansion to meet the needs of a growing community had by now become an ongoing managerial policy. Those who took over leadership roles after his death proceeded in a manner which he would heartily have approved.

In 1947, Five South opened, bringing the hospital's capacity up to 330 beds and 75 bassinets.

An honor came to a staff member in 1949 which would had gladdened my father's heart. Herina Eklind, the hospital superintendent, was awarded the Pioneer Medal by the King of Sweden for her work in connection with Swedish Hospital.

Modernization of the Tumor Institute took place in 1954, with the addition of a two million volt radiation tube and structural changes to provide the shielding it required. By then the Tumor Institute had become widely recognized both here and abroad. Patients came from all parts of the Northwest and Alaska to be treated there, and staff members made valuable contributions to cancer research through articles and books they published. The Tumor Institute also began to play an important role in attracting interns to train at Swedish, Hospital.

1954 saw the retirement of Miss Eklind, and the beginning of construction of the Doctor N.A. Johanson Wing, which was completed in 1955 at a cost of almost two million dollars. The new wing included space for laundry service, storage facilities, and administrative quarters. The following year the first three floors of the Johanson Wing (the west wing) were completed, bringing the capacity to 365 beds. A new level entrance and lobby were included, changing the hospital's main entrance from Summit to Columbia.

As every new project to improve the hospital was completed, I could almost hear my father saying, "Good! Just what we needed. Now here's what we should do next." He could always think of ways in which hospital services could be improved, and after his death those in charge continued in this farsighted attitude.

One addition to the hospital is particularly close to my heart. In 1955 my husband donated the Katharine Johanson Memorial Chapel to the hospital, in honor of my mother. It is open at all times to those in need of the quiet and solace which it offers. Hospital visitors often are involved in frightening or sad experiences as relatives or friends fight for life in the intensive care unit, or live out the final hours of a debilitating illness. At times like this a quiet place for prayer or meditation can be such a blessing. There is an adjoining family room for those whose spiritual beliefs may be centered in other than the Christian church. When Elmer decided to provide funds to build a chapel, I was touched that he wanted to dedicate it to my mother's memory. During the years it has been in existence I have heard many times from staff and visitors that the chapel is deeply appreciated.

I received the following letter from The Rev. Richard E. Johnson, who served as the hospital's chaplain for many years. I really appreciated his taking the time to tell me of all that the chapel has meant to patients, families and staff:

"Dear Mrs. Nordstrom:

It seemed good to me to take a few minutes and let you know how much I appreciate the chapel and family room at Swedish Hospital. It is used by patients and family members for meditation and prayer. I also see hospital personnel using it in the same way.

It has been good to have it when a family is suddenly bereaved and needs a place to express the first rush of grief in private. I have noticed that some of the physicians use it to talk with family members facing important decisions. It has also been used to have communion during Holy Week and Christmas Week. We have used it for memorial services when President Eisenhower died and when Robert Kennedy was shot. I have also had the privilege of conducting weddings in the chapel. It has known tears and the sound of weeping and joy and the sound of laughter.

So you can see that your memorial gift in behalf of your mother, Mrs. Johanson, continues to meet a very important spiritual-human need here at Swedish Hospital. Thank you most sincerely."

One of the chapel's more unusual weddings took place when a commercial fisherman from Alaska was married one week after he had triple bypass surgery. His coronary surgery recovery nurse served as an attendant, and his surgeons were guests of honor. At the reception which followed, a hospital wash basin doubled as a punch bowl and the dietary department provided a beautifully decorated wedding cake. The groom and his doctors were heard planning an Alaskan fishing trip together for the following summer.

In 1961 there were two important developments. One of these was the arrival of Dr. Allan Lobb as the hospital's medical director. He later was named exec-utive director, and in that position his wealth of talents and aggressive spirit of leadership were to have an immense impact on the institution's progress.

1961 was also the year that the Northwest Kidney Center was established at Swedish, although it later became a separate institution. With the invention of the artificial kidney by Dr. Belding Scribner of the University of Washington, the need for a special kidney center became apparent, and the Board of Directors of Swedish Hospital voted to offer the hospital as a site for this important work. It was initially established in Eklind Hall.

The fourth and fifth floors of the Johanson Wing were completed in 1962, and 1963 saw the addition of a sixteen room operating pavilion. In 1967 the sixth, seventh, eighth and ninth floors were added to the west wing, increasing capacity to 460 beds.

I know my father would have been particularly pleased at the hospital's association with the Fred Hutchinson Cancer Research Center, because of his deep interest in the battle against cancer.

The Center was founded in 1965 and named in honor of the prominent Seattle baseball star who died of cancer in 1964. Father's good friend, Doctor William Hutchinson, was Fred Hutchinson's older brother. He was primarily responsible for bringing this valued institution into being, and almost singlehandedly obtained the initial research grants and contracts with which the independent, nonprofit institution was funded. He served as its first director, from 1965 to 1984. The Fred Hutchinson Cancer Research Center has an international reputation, and performs more bone marrow transplants than any other institution in the world.

An indication of the quality of work performed at the Center is the 1990 award of the Nobel Prize to Doctor E. Donnall Thomas, founding director of its division of clinical research, for his pioneering work in the area of bone marrow transplants.

The relationship between "The Hutch," as it is often referred to, and Swedish has been very close. Bone marrow transplant patients from the Center are cared for at Swedish. The hospital has made a considerable investment in the special rooms and techniques which are needed to provide the sterile atmosphere required by these patients, who are extremely susceptible to infection during the transplant period.

In 1968 the Board made the decision to change the name from Swedish Hospital to Swedish Hospital Medical Center. This really was more appropriate in view of the many additional services now being offered to the community. In recent years the name was again changed, to Swedish Medical Center.

The big news for the decade of the 80's was of course the merging of Swedish Hospital, Doctors Hospital and Seattle General Hospital. The many years of planning which preceded the actual merger in 1980 required an incredible amount of patience and compromise on the part of the Boards for all three hospitals. Dr. Allan Lobb's role in orchestrating this entire procedure in an amicable atmosphere cannot be underestimated. The kind of imaginative and aggressive leadership which Dr. Lobb demonstrated during his twenty-seven years at Swedish is very much akin to my father's style of management. Dr. Lobb has been quoted as saying that all the progress he was able to achieve during his tenure was based directly on my father's foresight in establishing the Tumor Institute in 1932.

In 1985 Swedish Medical Center celebrated an important anniversary. Seventy-five years had gone by since that small group of dedicated Swedish immigrants determinedly pursued a goal which was to provide their adopted city with an outstanding medical facility. Swedes are sometimes said to be stubborn. Thank heaven for the stubbornness of my father and his friends, and their dogged insistence that Seattle would have a first-class hospital. What a heritage each of those men left! I'm sure all of their descendants must feel the same glow of pride which I experience when I think of my father's part in this enterprise.

I'm very proud also of the role my husband played in guiding the progress of this great institution. He was the only person to have been elected to sixteen consecutive terms on the board, and he served as president of the board seven times. As part of the seventy-fifth anniversary celebration. Elmer Nordstrom and Doctor William Hutchinson were awarded the Health Care Leadership Plaque.

Also announced at the anniversary celebration was the forthcoming construction of the Nordstrom Medical Tower, named in Elmer's honor. This is a professional condominium building, completed in 1986 at a cost of twenty million dollars. It provides 176,000 sq. ft. of office space for purchase or lease by physicians. I'm so glad this gesture of appreciation took place while Elmer was still with us.

There's a fine oil painting of Elmer in the lobby, done by a talented Los Angeles painter named Margaret Sargent. Elmer refused to sit for the portrait (just as my father refused to sit for his portrait that hangs in the main lobby at Swedish) so the artist had to work from photographs. Miss Sargent paints on linen, and we were very pleased with Elmer's portrait. Unfortunately there was some water damage to the lobby of the Elmer Nordstrom Tower shortly after it opened. Elmer's portrait got soaked, and the paint peeled right off the linen, so the artist had to get out the photographs and start all over. The second portrait is in place now. I'm so glad I didn't persist in trying to get Elmer to pose for the first portrait, because I know that even if I had succeeded, he never would have agreed to go through that a second time.

Many activities were included in the anniversary celebration. A call went out for all babies who had been born at Swedish, Doctors, Seattle General, or Maynard (which had been absorbed earlier by Seattle General). There was a response from 3,200 "babies," seventy-five of whom were chosen for special honor in the program. One of those was Gordon Parks, who was born in the hospital elevator. Suzanne Bell, another respondee, returned to the hospital as an adult to undergo a kidney transplant, which enabled her to lead a normal life. Several years later she gave birth to a baby at Swedish Hospital. One of the youngest participants at the seventy-fifth birthday party was Corrigan Logan, a baby who viewed the festivities from his mother's arms. His name deserves some explanation: In 1938 Douglas Corrigan, an amateur airplane pilot, achieved fame when news stories dubbed him "Wrong-way Corrigan." He gained this title by filing a flight plan to fly from New York to Los Angeles, and somehow ending up in Dublin, Ireland, instead. Corrigan Logan's name was bestowed upon him by his mother's obstetrician, the infant having arrived in this world by means of a breech birth.

And of course Swedish Hospital's own special baby, David Ishii, who spent his first three years as the delight of the hospital's nursing staff, was another honored guest.

I've already told you about my friend Dorothy Ditlefsen, who retired in 1980 as head nurse at the Tumor Institute. Dorothy was born at Swedish in 1912, and she too was an honored guest at the Seventy-Fifth Anniversary celebration.

Another of the returning "Swedish babies" was Doctor Robert Bain, who served a term as the hospital's Chief of Staff. Doctor Bain's father, William Bain, was a partner with my cousin, Perry Johanson, in the architectural firm of Naramore, Bain, Brady and Johanson, and Doctor Bain's brother is currently a partner in that firm.

Doctor Dean Crystal is another prominent Seattle physician who was born at Swedish. He served on the hospital's surgical staff for many years.

Festivities at the anniversary celebration included a marching band and a Turn of the Century fashion show. Of particular interest to my family was the presentation of the Nils August Johanson Inspirational Award to the staff member who had demonstrated outstanding employee performance. I was very touched when I learned that this was to be an annual award in honor of my father. He was indeed the guiding spirit of Swedish Hospital during his lifetime, and to me this award symbolizes the fact that his influence lives on.

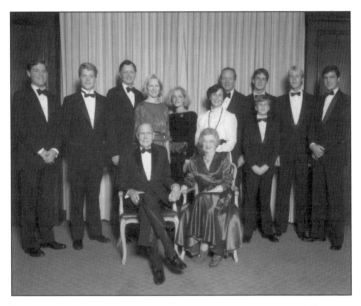

I love this family portrait, which was taken at our golden wedding anniversary celebration. Son John and his wife are standing behind Elmer. Son Jim and his wife and family are behind me. Aren't our grandchildren good-looking? I love them dearly.

Chapter Seventeen

Look What We Started!

I am grateful that my husband and I had such a long and happy marriage. We were married for almost 59 years. Elmer died in April of 1993 at Swedish Medical Center. Although there had been health problems from time to time, his final illness lasted only four days. I knew he was seriously ill, but his death still came as a shock, and I was grateful to have members of my family with me. Just as with my father's death, members of the hospital staff deeply felt the loss of one who had played such a large role in the medical center's success.

With the death of my beloved husband, memories came flooding back to me of our life together—our first date at the fraternity dance, the great enjoyment we took in our family, our vacations at Hood Canal, our travels abroad, the Seahawk years, and so on.

It didn't seem very long ago that Elmer and I had two lanky teen-agers around the house and a refrigerator with a swinging door. Jim and John are very successful business men now in the Nordstrom enterprises, but they were not always as enthusiastic about merchandising as they are today. My husband and his two brothers, Lloyd and Everett, began working in their father's shoe store at an early age. Our sons were given that same opportunity as youngsters, and seemed to enjoy it. When they were about eleven they worked in the stockroom, putting shoes away. They were paid 75 cents an hour.

By the time they were teen-agers, however, they sometimes had other ideas about how they would like to spend their summers. It wasn't that they didn't want to work. They just didn't want to work for the Nordstrom shoe stores (we had not yet entered the apparel business). For one thing, they didn't like the ribbing they took about being the boss's son.

One summer they each set out to prove they could make it on their own. (Remember young Kitty, determined to earn her own living at an early age?) John found a job pumping gas at Bryant's Marina, and Jim went to work in Swanson's nursery. One of them would come home covered with grease after his day's work, and the other would look pretty grubby after pushing wheelbarrows full of fertilizer or topsoil all day. By the next summer a nice clean shoe store looked really good to both of them, and that's how they chose to become involved in the Nordstrom enterprises rather than marinas and garden centers.

It might have been handy to have a marina in the family at that, since boating has been a big interest in our lives. Several years ago Elmer and I had our first cruise on the Northstream, a beautiful new 100 foot cruiser that Jim had built down in Westport. Any good Scandinavian will no doubt recognize that Northstream is the English translation of Nordstrom. It was the name which Elmer and I chose for the boat we owned.

We bought the original Northstream, a 34-foot ChrisCraft, in 1940. Just a year later came Pearl Harbor and our country's involvement in World War II. The rationing of gasoline made recreational boating all but impossible (unless you could depend on sail power). Elmer volunteered his services for one day a week and the use of his boat in the Coast Guard Auxiliary. It often turned out to be one night a week, and the assignment he drew was a bit worrisome for me. His duty was to anchor our boat outside the submarine net which was strung across the passage into Bremerton and contact any boat wishing to enter the harbor. With the wartime blackout I could think of just a lot of things that might go wrong out there on rough waters in the dark. No one knew at that time what plans the Japanese might have for Puget Sound.

At last the war was over and we could use the Northstream for happier pursuits. I loved those years when the boys were little and we spent many happy vacations on our boat. If I do say so myself I was a good crew member, and got to be quite expert at assisting the skipper in getting the boat through the locks. I also knew my way around the galley pretty well. My father enjoyed going out with us on the boat from time to time, as did Elmer's father, John W. Nordstrom. I am so grateful that when they were youngsters our sons knew and loved my father, and that as they were growing up

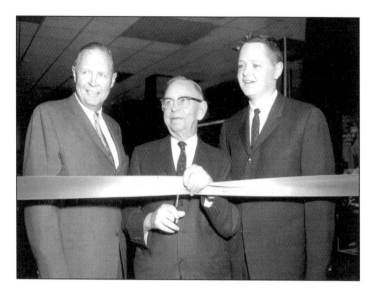

Three generations of Nordstroms: Our son John looks like a teen-ager here, but he was in his twenties and manager of the spokane Nordstrom shoe store. He joined his father and grandfather in this Grand Opening picture. The company founder, for whom John was named, was 91 when this was taken.

they also had a loving relationship with their Grandfather Nordstrom. He was a wonderful man, and lived to be 93 years old.

After the boys were on their own, Elmer and I continued to enjoy the Northstream. Elmer would take off several weeks in the summer so we could go on a cruise, and after he retired in 1970 we'd go up north for at least a month, sometimes longer. We knew lots of boating people. Wherever we'd go, when we'd reach a popular harbor there'd almost always be someone we knew. I loved it, because most of the time there'd be just the two of us on board. Several of our friends had boats, and sometimes we'd plan to meet somewhere. It was fun to pull into a quiet cove in the San Juans at dusk and anchor alongside our good friends the Donol Hedlunds on the Eugenie, or the Henry Bacons on the 4-B's.

I know that Jim and his family will have many happy years ahead of them aboard their Northstream. I'm glad to see my sons finding interests and activities outside their business, because they both work very hard and need some time of relaxation to balance their lives. In addition to boating, Jim really loves golf. John mainly likes to run. He used to run the 26 mile marathon. He ran the New York marathon three times, and the third time he ran it with his daughter, Kristin.

Each of our sons chose a lovely wife, and by chance they each married a girl named Sally, so we have Sally A. (nee Anderson), who is Jim's wife, and Sally B. (nee Boid), married to John. It gets a little confusing at times, but we're all used to it now.

Where have all the years gone? There are seven grandchildren and now there are seven great grandchildren as well! Seeing these wonderful little human beings become a part of our family gives me great joy and much to think about. In some of our younger ones I see a resemblance to my husband, and I think he saw something of me in others.

Now that most of our grandchildren are grown, as are the grandchildren of Everett and Lloyd, there are quite a few of that generation who are involved in the Nordstrom enterprises. I have to admit to some disappointment that none of my children or grandchildren have been at all interested in following a medical career.

Jim's wife, Sally A., is the daughter of Doctor William Anderson, a pediatrician, so I thought perhaps one of their boys would have some inclination toward a career in medicine, but it hasn't worked out that way.

It would be nice to have a young doctor in our family some day who could join the staff of Swedish Medical Center. Perhaps that will come with one of the great grandchildren. I know that my father would like to have had someone follow in his footsteps as a physician, because he wanted me to be a pediatrician. But on the other hand, wasn't he the one that said Swedes are such good businessmen? I'm very proud of the great success which my sons and their cousins and associates have made of the thriving business which they bought from Elmer and his brothers.

I have been asked if I see something of my father in my sons, and actually I do—not so much in appearance as in attitude. Much has been said about customer service being the reason for the tremendous success of the Nordstrom stores. I see some important parallels between the way my father managed his hospital, and the way my sons and their associates run the Nordstrom stores.

My father believed in choosing the most skilled persons he could find for his medical staff, and then supplying the very best of equipment for their work. He provided his nursing staff with good working conditions and with educational opportunities, and he stressed the importance of maintaining a pleasant attitude. He was often heard to tell them that it doesn't cost a thing to smile. He was never satisfied with status quo, but knew

LOOK WHAT WE STARTED!

the hospital must follow a pattern of planned growth—a tenet which the present management of Swedish Medical Center continues to espouse.

The methods my sons and their associates have used in achieving their great success are quite similar to those my father found effective in hospital management. Walk through any Nordstrom store and you will find employees who also have been made aware that a pleasant attitude means more sales for them and a happier time for the customer. These clerks work in attractive surroundings, and are given many educational opportunities to improve their skills. As for following a pattern of planned growth, this is quite evident with the succession of beautiful new Nordstrom stores which have appeared—each more innovative than the last. Members of the Nordstrom family are very excited at the prospect of a marvelous new flagship store which will emerge from the ashes, so to speak, of Frederick & Nelson. That should be a grand opening indeed and I won't even have to board a plane to attend!

I think what Father would have wanted for his grandsons was that they work hard to be the very best they could be, whether they chose the field of medicine, or merchandising, or any other worthwhile pursuit. He would have been particularly pleased that Jim and John N. Nordstrom and their business associates treat Nordstrom employees as if they were family members, which is the attitude my father always had toward his Swedish Hospital employees. It was the reason he was known affectionately to them as Papa Jo.

I am thankful our lives have been so rewarding and

that we have the inner resources to withstand any temporary troubles. I think back upon the many happy years I spent with Elmer and the wonderful family with which we have been blessed. Going back to earlier times, I am grateful for the happy childhood which my parents provided for me. That little girl who joyously rode horseback with her father or raced over the beach on Hood Canal doesn't seem too far beneath the layers of my life experience even now.

Katharine Johanson Nordstrom
Seattle, WA
1995

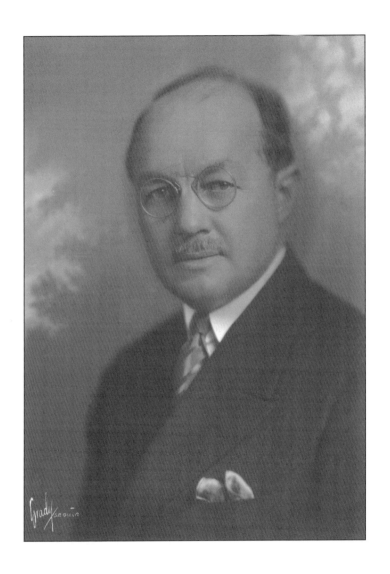

EPILOGUE

I never visit Swedish Medical Center without being reminded of my parents — there is the portrait of my father in the lobby, and the chapel dedicated to my mother's memory. When I see my husband's name on the Elmer Nordstrom Tower I think of the many years of leadership he contributed, a tradition of service carried on by our son Jim's participation on the Board.

I have so many memories connected with Swedish Medical Center— the birth of our sons, the serious illness of family members, the volunteer activities in which my family has participated, our friendship with staff members. The quest for excellence which was an integral part of my father's character lives on in the quality of care provided by this outstanding medical center.

Each of us makes whatever contribution we can to life while we are here. Very few of us are accorded the privilege of passing that contribution along for generations to come. My father was one of those fortunate few. The philosopher William James has said, "The greatest use of life is to spend it for something that outlasts it." Doctor Nils August Johanson spent his life in developing a medical facility which is a memorial to his courage, vision and dedication. I am very proud of his accomplishments, and especially grateful for my memories of him as a loving father.